Stem Cells in Cancer Treatment

Understanding the Science Behind a Breakthrough Approach

Marcio Alvarez-Silva, PhD

Stem Cells in Cancer Treatment: Understanding the Science Behind a Breakthrough Approach

ISBN n°978-65-01-68854-1

Cover art design by Marcio Alvarez-Silva

The Scientist Direct Publishing

Understanding Cancer
Learn to Win

To my wife, Adriana

"Wisdom is not a product of schooling but of the lifelong attempt to acquire it."

— Albert Einstein

Contents

Preface

> ***A Patient's Perspective:*** When Maria was diagnosed with a rare form of cancer, her world turned upside down. Chemotherapy was brutal, and surgery left her drained. But what bothered her was the feeling of uncertainty—not just about her chances of survival, but about whether there was anything else out there. She stumbled upon articles about stem cell therapy. *"Could it help me?"* She wondered. *"Is it real, or just hype?"*

This book is for Maria—and for all the people like her who are searching for answers.

In recent years, headlines have been filled with hopeful phrases like *"Stem Cells May Hold the Key to Curing Cancer"* or *"Breakthrough Therapies on the Horizon."* But what do these claims mean? How close are we to using stem cells as a reliable treatment for cancer? And more importantly, what does science say about this emerging field?

As researchers, doctors, and patients search for better, more precise, and less harmful ways to treat cancer, stem cells have emerged as one of the most promising tools in modern medicine. Their unique ability to develop into different types of cells and respond to signals in the body makes them intriguing candidates—not just for repairing damaged tissues, but for targeting cancer itself.

However, with promise comes complexity. There's a big gap between experimental studies in the lab and real-world therapies at the bedside. And in that space, myths, misunderstandings, and misinformation often spread.

That's the purpose of *Stem Cells in Cancer Treatment: What the Science Says About a Breakthrough Therapy.* This book is for everyone—patients, families, students, and anyone curious about the potential role of stem cells in the future of cancer care. You don't need a background in medicine or biology. Each chapter is designed to explain the science in simple, clear language, with illustrations and examples to help you along the way.

Hey there! I'm excited to share some insights into stem cells and their potential to revolutionize cancer treatment. We'll dive into the fascinating world of stem cells, understanding their functions and how cancer develops at the cellular level. We'll also explore the exciting developments in clinical trials and the ethical and safety concerns surrounding stem cell therapies. And guess what? We'll even peek into the future of stem cell research and its potential to prevent or even cure certain cancers.

Now, I know what you might be thinking: "Are these stem cell therapies miracle cures?" Well, not quite. But they're a promising avenue of hope for cancer patients like Maria and people like you. Stem cell therapies are still in the experimental stage, but they're making incredible progress and opening doors we never thought possible just a few decades ago. By understanding these developments, we can make better decisions, ask more informed questions, and feel more in control of our *learning journey*.

So, join me on this journey through one of the most fascinating and fast-moving frontiers in medical science. Together, we'll unravel the mysteries of stem cells and explore the potential of these incredible cells to transform the way we treat and prevent cancer.

Thanks for your time and curiosity. I look forward to sharing this journey with you!

Best regards,

Marcio Alvarez-Silva, PhD.

Introduction

Cancer is a major public health concern globally. It can be tough, making it hard to live a regular life. People with cancer go through a lot of emotions, and it's normal to feel scared, sad, angry, and powerless. You'll have good days and bad days, but with hard work and support, you can beat cancer and get better.

Each person's *cancer journey* is unique, and there's no one-size-fits-all approach. It can be a tough time, and it's okay to feel lonely or confused. But don't give up! With the proper support and treatment, you can overcome cancer.

Scientists are making great strides in treating cancer with new therapies. There are more effective medications with fewer side effects, and stem cell treatments are becoming more common.

Stem cells have shown great promise in cancer treatment, especially for leukemias and lymphomas. They've also been used to treat solid tumors like brain and breast cancer. In recent years, mesenchymal stem cells have been shown to have diverse therapeutic effects in treating various cancers and are becoming a crucial part of cancer treatment.

I invite you to explore this fascinating frontier of medicine with an open mind and a critical eye. The goal here is not to make promises, but to share what science genuinely tells us—and what it doesn't yet know—about one of the most compelling innovations in cancer research.

Part I: Understanding the Basics

Chapter 1 – What Are Stem Cells?

The Body's Master Builders

Every human being has an incredible self-repair system. If you cut your skin, it heals. If your blood cells get old, your body makes new ones. This amazing ability is thanks to something called ***stem cells.***

> ***Patient Quote:*** *"When my doctor first mentioned stem cells, I imagined something futuristic—like science fiction. I didn't realize they were already part of treatments saving lives today."* — Daniel, 35.

Stem cells are special because they don't have a specific job like blood cells or nerve cells do. Instead, they're **like blank tiles in a mosaic**. They can either remain blank and continue dividing (*self-renewal*) or change color and shape to fit into a specific part of the picture, such as skin, muscle, or blood—a process known as cell differentiation.

Stem cells are like little factories that can produce numerous copies of themselves. As they do this, they transform into different types of cells, each with a distinct function. This process is essential for the building and maintenance of all living things. It's like a recipe that tells cells what to become and how to work together. Scientists are still learning about how stem cells work and how to control them [1].

Cells in our bodies are like little workers with different jobs. For instance, hepatocytes reside in the liver, neurons are located in the brain, and red blood cells circulate through our veins. Each type of cell has its special skills and responsibilities. Hepatocytes are like the liver's bosses, making and sending bile, creating fats, and releasing special fats in the blood. Neurons are the brain's main workers, sending and receiving electrical and chemical messages that help us think and move. And red blood cells are like little oxygen delivery trucks, carrying oxygen to our tissues and taking away carbon dioxide.

This flexibility makes stem cells extremely important for human development, healing, and the development of new treatments for diseases such as cancer.

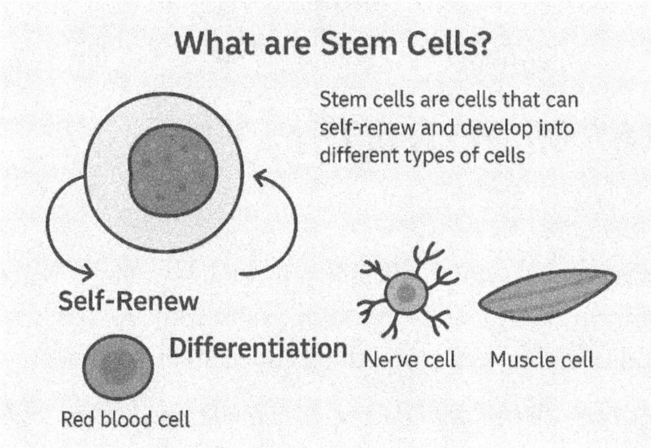

1.1 The Stem Cell Concept

Stem cells have come a long way since scientists first started studying them. In 1855, Robert Remak, a German scientist who studied embryonic development, made a groundbreaking discovery. According to Remak, the basic building blocks of life, called cells, come from the division of existing cells. [1]Rudolf Ludwig Carl Virchow (1821-1902) was a German physician, anthropologist, pathologist, biologist, writer, editor, and politician. In 1858, Rudolf Virchow made the famous saying "*omnis cellula e cellula*" (every cell comes from another cell) famous in a book called *Die Cellularpathologie* [2]. In 1858, Rudolf Virchow made the famous saying "*omnis cellula e cellula*" (every cell comes from another cell) famous in a book called *Die Cellularpathologie*. [3]. Back then, Virchow figured out that every living thing, whether it's a plant or an animal, is made up of tiny cells that come from other cells.

Diseases start in cells, which is why the Cell Theory states that all living things are composed of one or more cells. Cells are the basic building blocks of life, and they can only come from other cells.

To maintain the health of our organs and tissues, there are **a few key considerations to keep in mind.** First, we don't want the cells to grow too fast. Second, we don't want the number of cells to decrease. If they do, the organ or tissue can't function properly and starts to shrink or weaken. This can occur for various reasons and have serious consequences.

Stem cell research has been a hot topic in medicine for decades. We've learned a great deal about these remarkable cells, and now there are numerous exciting possibilities for utilizing them in medicine, particularly in regenerative medicine. The main goal is to fix damaged tissues and organs. This research has been beneficial in orthopedics, dermatology, and the treatment of chronic diseases. Stem cells are often utilized in conjunction with biomaterials, tissue engineering, and gene therapies. They've been used to treat conditions like spinal cord injuries, diabetes, neurodegenerative diseases, heart attacks, and bone fractures.

Stem cells in tissues typically remain dormant, neither growing nor maintaining high energy levels. However, when given the proper signal, they can resume growth. Scientists have observed this phenomenon in stem cells derived from various sources, including blood, hair follicles, muscles, and the brain. Differentiated cells don't continue to grow indefinitely. The balance between resting and growing stem cells must be carefully managed to prevent excessive cell growth in tissues. This helps maintain balance and aids in repairing damaged tissues.

Did You Know?
Stem cells are sometimes called the body's *"master cells"* because they can become more than 200 different types of cells—everything from muscle to nerve to blood.

1.2 Where Are Stem Cells Found?

You might be surprised to learn that stem cells exist in all of us—from the moment we are embryos to adulthood. Here's a breakdown of where they come from:

Embryonic Stem Cells (ESCs)

These are **early embryos**, just a few days after fertilization. ESCs are incredibly versatile because they can differentiate into *any* of the approximately 200 cell types found in the human body. Scientists use them extensively in basic research, but this comes with ethical concerns. Retrieving them usually means destroying the embryo. [4, 5].

Adult (Somatic) Stem Cells

These stem cells exist **within specific tissues** throughout the body. Their role is to maintain and repair those tissues as needed. They are **multipotent**, meaning they can differentiate into a limited range of cell types. Examples include:

- ***Hematopoietic Stem Cells (HSCs)*** – Found in bone marrow; they give rise to all blood cells.
- ***Neural Stem Cells*** – Found in the brain; they can produce certain types of neurons and glial cells.
- ***Epithelial Stem Cells*** – Help regenerate the lining of the gut and skin.
- ***Mesenchymal Stem Cells (MSCs)*** - Among the different types of adult stem cells, mesenchymal stem cells have garnered significant attention due to their ability to differentiate into various cell types. Friedenstein first identified these stem cells in the 1960s during his studies of bone marrow. [6]. Mesenchymal stem cells can be found in different adult tissues, not just bone marrow. They've been spotted in various tissues, including fat, dental pulp, placenta, amniotic fluid, umbilical cord blood, Wharton's jelly, brain, spleen, liver, kidney, lung, thymus, and pancreas.[7-13].

MSCs can differentiate into **bone, cartilage,** or **fat cells,** and they have a remarkable ability to **reduce inflammation** and **modulate the immune system.** These qualities make them a subject of intense interest in **cancer therapy** and **regenerative medicine** [14-18].

Unlike ESCs, adult stem cells do not raise major ethical concerns and are already used in some approved treatments, such as **bone marrow transplants** for leukemia [19, 20].

Induced Pluripotent Stem Cells (iPSCs)

Discovered in 2006 by Dr. Kazutoshi Takahashi and Dr. Shinya Yamanaka, iPSCs are **adult cells that have been reprogrammed** to behave like embryonic stem cells. This technique enables scientists to create pluripotent cells without using embryos, offering a robust and **ethically acceptable alternative** [21].

Did You Know?
Embryonic stem cells were first successfully grown in a laboratory in **1998**, a milestone that marked the beginning of modern stem cell research.

1.3 Let's dive into the main types of adult stem cells.

Hematopoietic Stem Cells

Hematopoietic stem cells (HSCs) are special cells that make all the blood and immune cells in our bodies. They primarily reside in the bone marrow and can continue to divide and differentiate into various types of blood cells, including red blood cells, white blood cells, and platelets. These cells are like little factories that produce all the blood and immune cells we need throughout our lives. They're highly essential to maintaining the health of our blood and immune systems. In fact, the first time stem cells were used in cancer treatment was back in 1957. Scientists studied five patients with leukemia and one patient with ovarian cancer who got total body radiation and chemotherapy. They then gave these patients blood stem cells from a healthy donor. The scientists examined different doses of stem cells and the time it took for patients to recover. They also wanted to know if the stem cells could help patients return to their normal health. [22].

Stem cells from healthy donors were used in the procedure, making bone marrow transplantation a rapidly popular treatment. It uses hematopoietic stem cells to treat various medical conditions. Bone marrow transplantation was first used to treat people with inherited immune problems, bone marrow failure, and cancer.

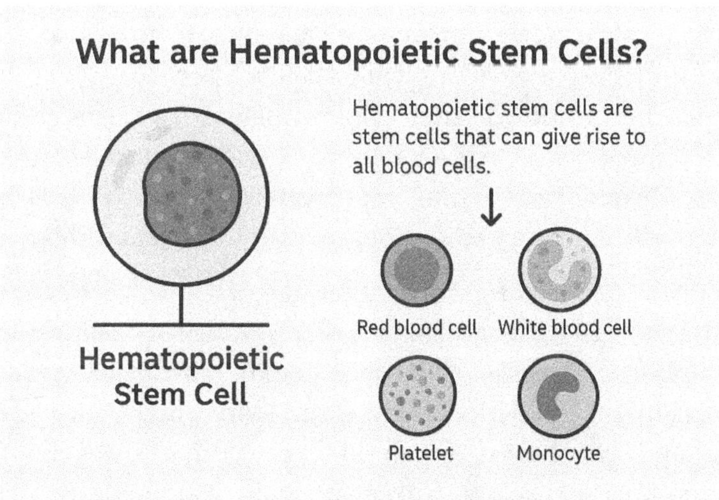

In the 1980s and 1990s, advancements in *in vitro* cell propagation techniques and enhancements in the procedures associated with transplantation led to a significant increase in the number of transplants. Consequently, both national and international bone marrow registries were established.

HSCs were traditionally obtained from bone marrow, which is why this type of transplant was called a **bone marrow transplant**. However, thanks to new methods for isolating stem cells from alternative sources, such as peripheral blood or umbilical cord blood, we now refer to it as a **hematopoietic stem cell transplant**.

When the procedure started, they took bone marrow samples from both hips to obtain sufficient bone marrow. As time went on, with advancements in stem cell biology and the development of specialized drugs, stem cell transplants became increasingly easier. Now, most of the procedures in adults (more than 70%) use stem cells from a donor's blood. [20].

HSC transplantation is a standard procedure used in cancer treatment centers worldwide. It's like giving your body a blood transfusion, but instead of blood, it provides you with stem cells that can help your body make new blood and immune cells. This is especially helpful for people who have been through a lot of chemotherapy or radiation, which can make it hard for their bodies to fight off infections and diseases.

There exist two principal types of hematopoietic stem cell transplantation:

1. **Autologous hematopoietic stem cell transplantation** is a process where the patient's own blood cells are collected before starting primary treatment, which might include chemotherapy and radiation. These cells are then kept safe in a lab or frozen for later infusion after treatment. This helps to restore the patient's blood and immune systems.
2. **Allogeneic hematopoietic stem cell transplantation** means getting stem cells from someone who's not a family member. You can collect these stem cells while you're already getting your treatment. This way, you have the stem cells ready right away, so you can get your transplant without issues.

Hematopoietic stem cell transplantation was first used to treat leukemia, but it's also used to treat autoimmune diseases, such as multiple sclerosis, Crohn's disease, and sickle cell anemia. [23-26]. Most hematopoietic stem cell transplants are still performed to treat blood cancers, such as multiple myeloma and lymphoma, which are the primary reasons for cell transplants. Acute myeloid leukemia, acute lymphoblastic leukemia, myelodysplastic syndromes, and myeloproliferative neoplasms are the main reasons for allogeneic hematopoietic stem cell transplantation. Transplantation can also be used to treat other types of tumors, like germ cell tumors, neuroblastoma, Ewing's sarcoma, and medulloblastoma. [24, 25].

Stem cell grafts show promise in treating various types of cancer. However, they're expensive and require a significant amount of preparation for patients. So, doctors are looking for other ways to treat solid tumors without the intense conditioning.

Did You Know?
Bone marrow transplants have saved lives since the **1960s.**

Mesenchymal Stem Cells

Mesenchymal stem cells (MSCs) are multipotent stromal cells that possess the capability to differentiate into various cell types, including osteoblasts, adipocytes, and chondrocytes. These cells were initially isolated from bone marrow by Friedenstein et al. [13] in the 1970s. MSCs have emerged as a focal point in the field of regenerative medicine, owing to their ease of isolation, immunomodulatory properties, and their potential to facilitate tissue repair and regeneration. Over the past several decades, advancements in the field of stem cell biology have positioned MSCs at the forefront of both translational and clinical research.

Although bone marrow serves as the source of MSCs, various tissues have since been identified as viable sources:

- **Bone marrow**: This traditional source exhibits a low frequency of MSCs, approximately 0.001% to 0.01% of cells.
- **Adipose tissue**: This tissue offers a higher yield of MSCs through minimally invasive procedures [27].
- **The umbilical cord**, which includes Wharton's jelly and cord blood, provides immunologically naive MSCs [28].
- **The placenta**, **dental pulp**, **synovial membrane**, and **amniotic fluid** serve as alternative sources that enhance accessibility and applicability [29-32].

MSCs are like the body's repair crew. They can change into different types of tissues, like bone, fat, and cartilage. This makes them super helpful in healing and growing new tissue. But how do scientists know they're dealing with real MSCs instead of other cells? Well, the International Society for

Cellular Therapy (ISCT) has established guidelines to ensure they're on the right track. [33]:

1. *MSCs adhere to plastic when cultivated in vitro.* When grown in the laboratory under standard conditions, MSCs naturally adhere to plastic culture plates. This characteristic serves as one of the initial indicators scientists utilize to identify them.
2. *MSCs possess a unique "ID badge".* They exhibit specific proteins on their surface that function as identification tags. These proteins are readily identifiable and include CD105, CD73, and CD90. Conversely, they do not express the proteins typically associated with blood-forming cells, such as CD45 and CD34. It is noteworthy that the CD34 protein is characterized in hematopoietic stem cells.
3. *MSCs can differentiate into three principal types of tissue-forming cells.* Within the laboratory setting, MSCs must substantiate their ability to transform into bone cells (osteoblasts), adipose cells (adipocytes), and cartilage cells (chondrocytes). This versatility is a fundamental aspect of their classification as stem cells.

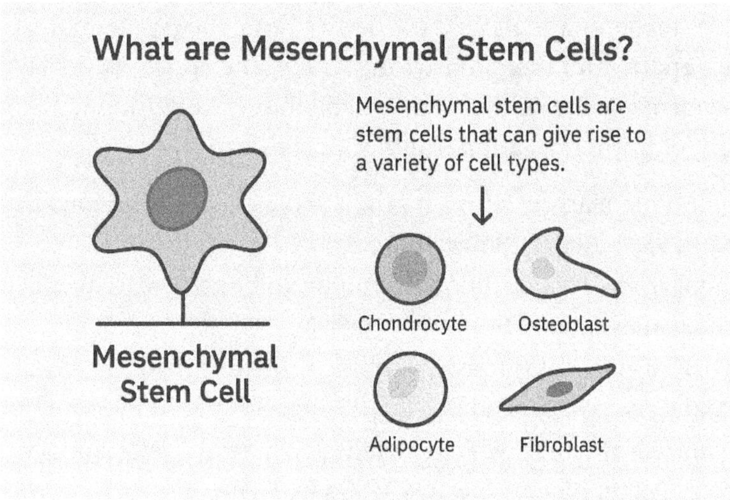

These guidelines help researchers worldwide ensure they are working with the same type of cell. It is akin to possessing an international recipe that defines what constitutes a true MSC. By adhering to these criteria, scientists can compare results and develop therapies that are both reliable and reproducible.

The most significant capabilities of MSCs arise from their ability to communicate with other cells and influence the healing process. The following outlines the three primary ways in which mesenchymal stem cells contribute to the body's healing process [34, 35].

MSCs differentiation: The process of transforming into new cell types

This is the initial concept that individuals often associate with the term "stem cells." MSCs possess the ability to differentiate into bone, adipose (fat), or cartilage cells [33]. If an individual has a damaged bone or joint, MSCs may assist by transforming into new tissue. However, current research indicates that this is not the primary mechanism through which MSCs contribute to the body; rather, it constitutes merely one aspect of a larger framework.

MSCs Cellular Signaling: Sending Helpful Messages

MSCs can assist many cells in different tissues by emitting minute chemical signals. These signals serve as messages that instruct other cells on their appropriate actions. Notably, MSCs can:

1. Prevent cells from dying in injured areas.
2. Stimulate the existing cells to repair themselves.
3. Facilitate the growth of new blood vessels through protein signals that act as "local hormones," such as Vascular Endothelial Growth Factor (VEGF)[1].
4. Decrease inflammation by releasing anti-inflammatory proteins such as Interleukin 10 (IL-10)[2] .

Consider MSCs as managers at a construction site; they do not engage in all the labor themselves, but rather coordinate the efforts of others to accomplish the task at hand [35].

The *in vitro* cultivation of MSCs is crucial for clinical-scale applications. The accessibility and the quantity of stem cells obtained vary according to the source. For instance, adipose tissue yields a greater number of MSCs than does bone marrow. In contrast, umbilical cord-derived MSCs are

---

1Have you heard of VEGF? It's a super important protein that helps blood vessels grow and heal. It's like a messenger that tells the cells lining blood vessels to grow and multiply.

2IL-10 is a protein molecule called a *cytokine. It's like a superhero* that fights inflammation and helps keep our immune system in check. It does this by telling the immune system to chill out and not overreact to bad guys, so our bodies don't get hurt and stay healthy.

regarded as more "primitive cells" and may possess enhanced proliferative potential [14, 36].

Immunomodulation: Controlling the Immune System

MSCs demonstrate particular efficacy in circumstances where the immune system exhibits excessive reactivity. They possess the ability to: 1) inhibit the overactivity of specific immune cells, such as T cells; 2) enhance the proliferation of regulatory cells that maintain equilibrium within the immune system; and 3) diminish the activity of cells responsible for inflammation. Consequently, MSCs prove beneficial in the management of autoimmune diseases, wherein the body erroneously targets its own tissues, as well as in conditions such as severe infections or transplant rejection, where regulating the immune response is of paramount importance [34].

Together, these three functions—differentiation, signaling, and immune regulation—render MSCs powerful instruments for facilitating healing and recovery across a broad spectrum of medical conditions.

1.4 What Makes Stem Cells So Valuable?

Stem cells are valuable for three key reasons:

1. They Are a Natural Repair System

Whenever tissue is damaged—due to injury, disease, or age—stem cells may activate to replace or restore it. This natural regenerative capacity is being harnessed to treat **degenerative diseases**, burns, and even spinal cord injuries.

2. They Help Us Understand Disease

By studying how stem cells become specialized, scientists can learn what goes wrong during diseases like cancer or Parkinson's. Stem cells allow us to watch development unfold in a dish—something we could never do in a living person.

3. They're Tools for Drug Discovery and Testing

Instead of testing drugs on animals or patients, scientists can grow stem cells in the lab and test new compounds in a controlled environment, reducing risk and cost.

1.5 The Link Between Stem Cells and Cancer

At first glance, stem cells and cancer cells might seem like opposites—one heals, the other harms. However, they share some similarities in fact. Both can self-renew and multiply. This has led to the discovery of **cancer stem cells**—a subset of tumor cells that may drive tumor growth, resistance to treatment, and relapse [37].

Researchers are also investigating how **healthy stem cells** can be used to **seek out tumors**, deliver anti-cancer agents, or stimulate the immune system to fight back. For example, MSCs may be engineered to carry therapeutic genes into tumors, acting like a biological "**Trojan horse**".

1.6 Misconceptions and Realities

Due to their powerful potential, stem cells have been surrounded by hype—and, unfortunately, misinformation. Some private clinics market unproven stem cell treatments to desperate patients, claiming to treat everything from Amyotrophic Lateral Sclerosis (ALS) to cancer. These treatments often lack evidence, are **not approved by regulatory agencies**, and may pose serious health risks [38].

If you're considering any stem cell-based therapy, it's essential to check whether:

- It is part of a registered clinical trial.
- It has **published results** in peer-reviewed journals.
- It is approved by **regulatory authorities** (such as the EMA, FDA, or ANVISA).

This book will help you learn to distinguish between **experimental therapy, proven therapy**, and **unregulated treatment**.

1.7 A Glimpse into the Future

Scientists are only beginning to unlock the full potential of stem cells. What we know today is just a fraction of what we'll know in 10 or 20 years. From growing new organs to curing genetic diseases, the future holds numerous possibilities for prosperity.

In the chapters ahead, you'll see how stem cells are being developed specifically to combat cancer—from **rebuilding immune systems after**

chemotherapy to **attacking tumors directly**. We'll examine what's real, what's experimental, and what's on the horizon.

Chapter 2 – Cancer: A Disease of the Cells

Cancer is one of the most feared diseases in the world. But what exactly is it?

> ***Patient Quote:*** *"When I was diagnosed, I kept asking myself: how did my own cells turn against me? Learning about how cancer starts helped me understand what was happening inside my body."* – Rosa, 52.

Cancer is a condition in which specific cells in the body cease to follow the standard rules of growth. Instead of growing, dividing, and dying in an orderly manner, these cells continue to multiply without control. Over time, they can form lumps called **tumors** and, in some cases, travel to other parts of the body.

Unlike healthy cells, which work together to keep the body functioning, cancer cells act independently, ignoring the signals that tell them to stop growing. This uncontrolled behavior is what makes cancer harmful – it can damage organs, tissues, and the body's natural balance.

At its core, cancer is a disease that begins in our own cells. It occurs when the standard rules that govern how cells grow and behave begin to break down. As a result, cells start to grow out of control, and this can lead to the formation of a lump or tumor. Some of these cancer cells can break away from the tumor and spread to other parts of the body through the blood vessels or lymphatic system. In this case, there is a risk of the disease growing in different parts of the body, which increases the risk of cancer.

__Patient Story – Meet Hellen:__ "I was 41 when I found a small lump under my arm. I thought it was nothing. But tests showed it was breast cancer. I remember sitting in the hospital waiting room, overwhelmed. I didn't know anything about cancer. Learning how it starts in the cells helped me understand what was happening inside my body."

Did You Know?
Cancer is not a single disease—there are **more than 200 types of cancer**, each with different causes, behaviors, and treatments.

2.1 What Do Healthy Cells Do?

Our bodies are made up of trillions of cells that work together to keep us alive and healthy. Each cell has a specific function, and they work together to form tissues and organs that keep our bodies alive and functioning. Cells usually grow, divide to make new cells, and then die when they're no longer needed. This entire process helps keep our bodies in balance. It's like a well-run city where buildings are built when needed and old ones are safely removed. When it's time for a cell to die, it goes through a process called **apoptosis**, or programmed cell death. Apoptosis eliminates cells that aren't functioning correctly or are in excess. This way, the growth of cells in our organs and tissues is carefully controlled.

Every time a cell divides, it must make an exact copy of its DNA, which serves as the body's instruction manual for life. This "manual" has all the info needed to keep your body running smoothly.

Helpful Analogy
DNA is like the software that runs a cell. If the software becomes corrupted, the cell can behave like a malfunctioning machine—reproducing when it shouldn't, avoiding shutdown, and ignoring safety limits.

Every cell in your body carries a complete set of **chromosomes**, which are like neatly packed bookshelves holding your DNA. You can think of this DNA as a tiny instruction manual inside each cell—it tells the cell how to grow, when to divide, and even when it's time to shut down in a safe, controlled process called **apoptosis**. This built-in recycling system removes old or damaged cells, allowing fresh, healthy ones to take their place.

Imagine zooming in on DNA. You'll see it's like a twisted ladder, called the double helix. The "rungs" are made up of chemical building blocks, like letters in a special code (A, T, C, and G). These sequences form **genes, like chapters in an instruction manual**. Each gene provides the cell with instructions to produce **proteins**, which perform most of the work necessary to keep us alive and healthy.

What Is a Gene?

A gene is a tiny part of your body's instruction manual, the DNA. It tells your body how to grow, work, and stay healthy. Genes, made of DNA, give instructions to make proteins, which do almost everything your body needs —like building muscles, digesting food, and fighting off infections.

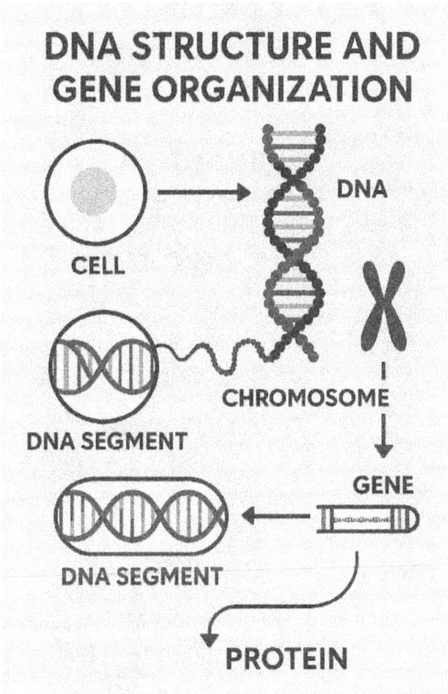

Why Are Genes Important?

- They control how your body develops and functions.
- They help repair your body when you're hurt or sick.
- They play a role in how you respond to food, medicine, and your environment.

Typically, your body has natural "proofreading" systems that identify and correct errors in DNA. But sometimes, small mistakes slip through. These changes, known as **mutations**, can occur in genes. Most mutations are harmless or quickly repaired. But if a mutation occurs in a gene that makes a critical **protein controlling cell growth**, that protein may no longer work properly. A faulty protein can act like a broken traffic light—sending the wrong signals or no signals at all. When this happens, cells may start dividing too quickly or ignore the usual "stop" signals, which can lead to cancer or other diseases.

If mutations happen and are not repaired, the cell may not work correctly. Most of the time, these errors are harmless and are typically corrected by the body. But sometimes, a single mistake can lead to cancer later on.

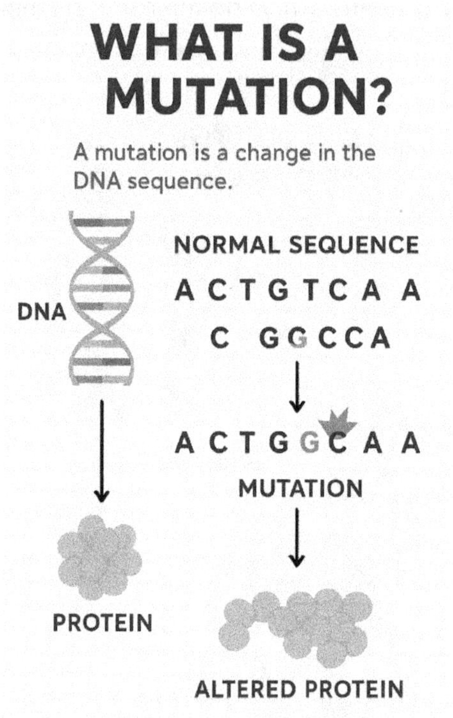

Did You Know?
Your body makes billions of new cells every day. Sometimes, minor "typos" in the DNA instructions—called **mutations**—can happen, and these can occasionally lead to cancer.

2.2 Where do Mutations Come From?

Mutations can happen for many reasons, and cancer often develops from a combination of genetic conditions and environmental factors [39-42].

Inherited Mutations (Genetic Factors)

Some people are born with specific gene mutations that increase their risk of developing cancer. These inherited mutations are passed down from a parent and are present in every cell of the body from birth.

Examples include mutations in the ***BRCA1*** and ***BRCA2*** genes, which raise the risk of breast and ovarian cancers. Another example is **Lynch syndrome**, which increases the risk of colon and endometrial cancers. However, inherited mutations are responsible for only about 5–10% of all cancers.

Acquired Mutations (Environmental and Lifestyle Factors)

Most mutations develop during a person's lifetime and are not inherited. These are known as **acquired mutations**, which arise from DNA damage caused by routine exposures or actions.

Common causes of acquired mutations include [41, 42]:

- **Tobacco smoke** is a significant cause of lung, throat, and mouth cancers.
- **Ultraviolet (UV) radiation from the sun** is the leading cause of skin cancer.
- **Certain viruses,** such as human papillomavirus (HPV), are linked to cervical and other cancers.
- **Exposure to harmful chemicals**, such as asbestos or industrial toxins, can be detrimental to health.
- **Unhealthy lifestyle choices**, including a poor diet, obesity, and a lack of exercise, can lead to various health issues.

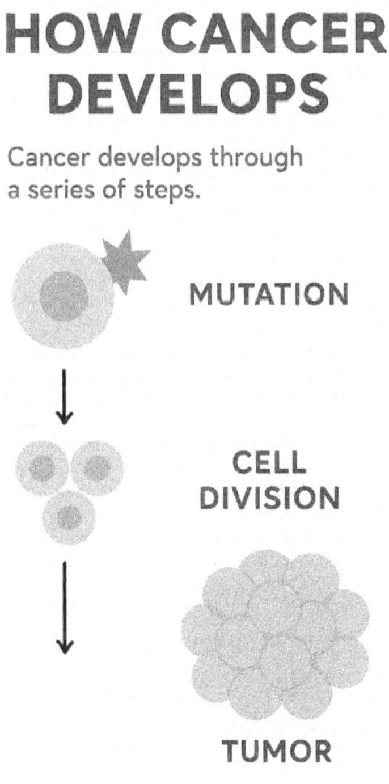

Key Facts

- A mix of genetic, environmental, and lifestyle factors causes cancer (National Cancer Institute) [38].
- Tobacco use alone is responsible for roughly 30% of all cancer deaths worldwide [34, 35].

2.3 It is Not Just One Mutation—It is Many

Cancer does not happen from a single mutation. It usually **takes multiple genetic changes over time** for a normal cell to become cancerous. That's why cancer is more common as people age—cells have had more time to accumulate genetic errors in DNA.

As these changes build up, cells may gain several dangerous abilities [43-45]:

- Grow without limits.
- Ignore signals to stop dividing.
- Avoid being destroyed by the immune system.
- Recruit blood vessels to feed itself.
- Spread to other parts of the body (metastasis).

This gradual transformation from a normal cell into a cancer cell can take years—and during much of that time, the person may feel completely healthy. That's why it's crucial to recognize even the slightest signs that something is off.

Key Facts

- Over 10 million people are diagnosed with cancer each year worldwide (World Health Organization) [37].

2.4 Cancer Is Not "One Thing"

Because every person's DNA is different, and each cancer develops from a unique mix of genetic changes, no two cancers are exactly alike. That's why cancer treatment is becoming more personalized—what works for one patient might not work for another.

Over time, these abnormal cells can accumulate and form a lump or mass known as a tumor. Tumors are divided into two main types:

1. **Benign tumors**: These are non-cancerous. They may grow in size, but do not spread to other parts of the body. They can often be removed and are not usually life-threatening.

2. **Malignant tumors:** These are cancerous. They can invade nearby tissues, damage organs, and spread to distant parts of the body through the blood or lymphatic system. This process is called *metastasis*.

Not all cancers form tumors. Some types, like leukemia, begin in the bone marrow and affect the blood. These cancerous cells circulate throughout the body and interfere with the production of healthy blood cells, even though no solid tumor is formed.

Cancer can pop up in almost any part of your body, like in the lungs, breasts, colon, prostate, skin, or blood. And guess what? Each type of cancer is like a unique character with its special moves. They all have one thing in common: they grow out of control, but they can spread at different speeds, and they respond to treatment differently, varying in severity.

One of the most important things to know is that *cancer is treatable*—and often curable—especially when detected early. Thanks to decades of research, many people now survive cancer and live long, healthy lives after diagnosis.

Today, doctors can often test a tumor's genetic makeup to choose treatments that are more likely to work for that specific type of cancer. This is known as *precision medicine*.

> *Helpful Analogy*
> Think of your cells like cars in traffic. In a healthy body, they stop at red lights, go when it's safe, and follow the rules. Cancer cells are like reckless drivers who ignore all the signs—they speed, crash into others, and go wherever they want.

2.5 How Does Cancer Start?

Cancer begins deep within the body—often long before any symptoms appear—when something goes wrong in a single cell. Cancer doesn't happen all at once. It usually develops over time through a series of steps:

1. **Initiation** – A cell gets a mutation in its DNA.
2. **Promotion** – That cell begins to grow and divide more than it should.
3. **Progression** – The abnormal cell becomes more aggressive and begins to spread.

Over time, cancer cells can grow together into a mass called a **tumor,** which is like an unwanted lump of rapidly dividing cells. What makes cancer especially dangerous is that some of these cells can break away, travel through the bloodstream or lymphatic system, and migrate to new locations in the body. This spreading process is called **metastasis**, and it's how cancer can move from one organ to another, making it harder to treat.

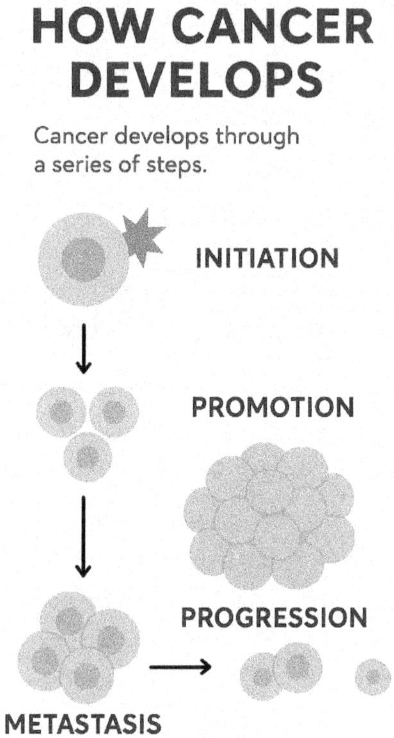

Helpful Analogy
Think of it like seeds carried by the wind that sprout far from the original plant—they can start growing again.

2.6 Genes That Play a Role in Cancer

Inside every cell are thousands of genes that tell it what to do. Some genes help the cell grow, while others instruct it when to stop. Cancer happens when specific genes go wrong:

- **Oncogenes** are like a gas pedal stuck down—making the cell grow too fast.
- **Tumor suppressor genes** are like brakes. When these are broken, the cell can't stop growing.

One essential gene is *p53*, known as the "*guardian of the genome.*" It helps detect when a cell's DNA is damaged and stops it from dividing. If p53 is not working, the cell can become dangerous [46].

2.7 The Traits of Cancer Cells

Scientists have discovered that, regardless of where cancer originates in the body, the cells often exhibit similar behavior. These shared traits are called the **hallmarks of cancer**. Think of them as the "common tricks" cancer cells use to survive and spread [43, 44]:

1. They grow when they shouldn't.
2. They don't listen to the signals to stop.
3. They avoid dying.
4. They keep dividing forever.
5. They create new blood vessels to feed themselves.
6. They can spread to other parts of the body.

By studying these hallmarks, researchers can gain a deeper understanding of what makes cancer so powerful and develop treatments that target its vulnerable areas.

> ***Patient Insight** – **Ana:** "When my doctor explained how cancer cells ignore signals to stop growing, it helped me see why treatment needs to be so strong—to stop something that refuses to stop on its own."*

Did You Know?

The word *cancer* comes from the Greek word for *crab*. Ancient doctors thought some tumors looked like crabs, with "legs" spreading out into nearby tissues—just as cancer can spread in the body. This image of a crab gripping and holding on gave the disease its name.

2.8 Cancer Isn't Just One Disease

Cancer is not just one disease, but a group of diseases that all involve a common problem: some of the body's cells begin to grow and divide out of control. These cells don't follow the standard rules that healthy cells obey —they ignore signals to stop growing, they avoid cell death to control the size of tissues, and they can spread to other parts of the body where they do not belong.

Each tumor isn't just made of one kind of cell—it's more like a mixed community of different cancer cells living together. Some of these cells grow very quickly, while others may be more resistant to standard treatments like chemotherapy or radiation. Hidden within this mix are often a smaller group of cells called **cancer stem cells (CSCs)**. These cells are special because they can "renew" themselves and create new cancer cells, much like how normal stem cells make healthy new cells in the body. Scientists believe CSCs may be one of the reasons why some cancers return even after treatment, because if these cells survive, they can rebuild the tumor later on [47].

> *Helpful Analogy*
> These cells are like the roots of a weed. You can cut the weed above ground, but if the root remains, it may grow again.

2.9 What Causes Cancer?

Many things can cause cancer. Some are out of our control, while others are related to our environment or lifestyle:

- **Inherited genes** from our parents (like BRCA mutations in breast cancer).
- **Tobacco smoking** is a significant cause of lung and other cancers.
- **Too much sun exposure** can damage skin cells.
- **Certain viruses**, such as human papillomavirus (HPV) or hepatitis B and C, are examples.
- **Poor diet**, lack of exercise, alcohol use, and obesity.

The World Health Organization's cancer research agency, the International Agency for Research on Cancer (IARC), has studied many of these risks and helps inform public health efforts worldwide [48].

2.10 How Doctors Diagnose and Treat Cancer

When doctors suspect cancer, they use tools like:

- **Scans** (CT, MRI, or PET) to look inside the body.
- **Biopsies** are taken to take a sample of tissue and check for cancer cells.
- **Genetic tests** to look for mutations that might guide treatment.

Treatment depends on the type of cancer and how advanced it is. Common treatments include:

- **Surgery** to remove the tumor.
- **Radiation therapy** destroys cancer cells with energy beams.
- **Chemotherapy** kills fast-growing cells.
- **Immunotherapy** to help the immune system fight cancer.

- **Targeted therapy** that blocks specific molecules in cancer cells that favor growth.
- **Stem cell therapy** is primarily used in the treatment of blood cancers.

No two people are alike, and neither are their cancers. Doctors now use **personalized medicine** to tailor treatments based on a person's genes and the biology of their tumor.

> ***Patient Reflection – Mary:*** *"I had to go through chemo, surgery, and radiation. It was tough. But when my oncologist explained the science behind each treatment, I felt more confident and in control."*

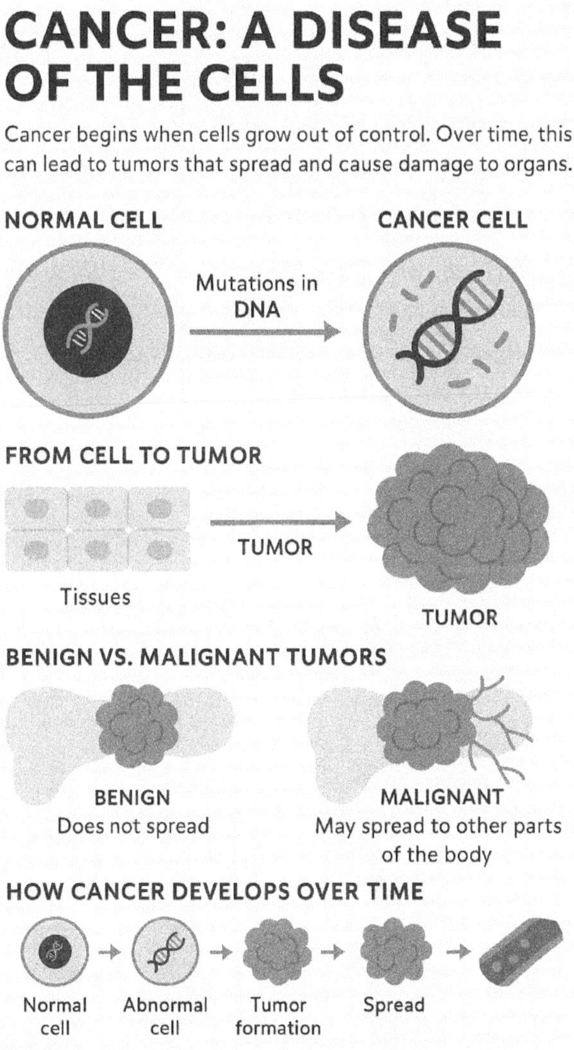

2.11 Why Learning About Cancer Helps Everyone

Cancer is a complex disease, but understanding its development and spread can make a significant difference for everyone. When we know the basics—how cells grow, what happens when they malfunction, and why tumors form—we are better equipped to take action. This may involve **getting regular screenings,** such as mammograms or colonoscopies, **making lifestyle choices** that reduce risk (like avoiding tobacco, eating healthier, and exercising), or simply knowing when to consult a doctor about concerning symptoms.

Knowledge also empowers us to be active participants in the fight against cancer. By staying informed, we can **support research** that leads to new therapies, advocate for improved healthcare policies, and stand by loved ones who are undergoing treatment. Even small actions, such as raising awareness in our communities, can have a ripple effect.

The more we understand, the better we can **prevent, detect, and treat** this disease—not just for ourselves, but for future generations.

In the next chapter, we will turn to stem cells—the body's remarkable **building blocks of life**—and see how they are giving scientists fresh tools to design better treatments, reduce side effects, and perhaps one day make cancer a disease we can truly cure.

Chapter 3 – Where Stem Cells and Cancer Meet

At first glance, stem cells and cancer might seem like two very different things—one brings hope for healing, while the other is a disease we fear. But in recent years, scientists have discovered essential ways in which these two biological forces are connected. Understanding the intersection between stem cells and cancer can help us better comprehend how cancer develops, why it sometimes recurs, and how new treatments may work in the future.

3.1 Stem Cells Characteristics

Stem cells are special cells in the body that have two key abilities:

1. **Self-renewal** – They can replicate themselves.
2. **Differentiation** – They can turn into many different types of specialized cells (like muscle cells, nerve cells, or blood cells).

Think of stem cells as the body's natural repair system. They reside in various tissues and are always ready to divide, helping to replace old or damaged cells. In fact, during early development in the womb, stem cells give rise to every organ and tissue in the body.

3.2 What Are Cancer Stem Cells?

In some cancers, scientists have identified a unique subset of cells that exhibit stem cell-like properties. These are known as **cancer stem cells (CSCs)**. Similar to normal stem cells, CSCs can self-renew and generate various types of cells found within a tumor. However, unlike healthy stem cells that contribute to tissue repair and regeneration, CSCs primarily give rise to more cancer cells, driving tumor growth and progression [47].

> ***Patient Quote:*** *"I had never heard of cancer stem cells before. My oncologist explained that they might be the reason some cancers come back, even after treatment. It made me realize why research is so important."* — Miguel, 47.

Researchers believe that CSCs may play several critical roles in the behavior of cancer:

- **Initiation**: CSCs may be responsible for the origin of certain types of cancer. Their capacity for self-renewal means that a single CSC can give rise to an entire tumor.
- **Tumor Growth**: CSCs can continuously produce cancer cells, fueling the expansion of the tumor mass.
- **Resistance to Treatment**: CSCs often survive traditional cancer therapies like chemotherapy and radiation, which mainly target rapidly dividing cells. CSCs may lie dormant or divide slowly, escaping destruction [49].
- **Recurrence and Metastasis**: After treatment, surviving CSCs can migrate to other parts of the body and seed new tumors, contributing to cancer relapse and spread [50].

Helpful Analogy

Think of CSCs like the roots of a weed. Even if the top is cut off (the visible tumor), the origins remain hidden in the soil. Without removing the roots, the weed can grow back. Similarly, cancer treatments that fail to eliminate CSCs may leave behind the seeds for future tumors.

Ongoing research aims to identify the molecular markers that distinguish CSCs from regular cells, such as surface proteins: CD133 in brain tumors or CD44 in breast cancers. This may allow doctors to develop therapies that specifically target CSCs while sparing healthy tissues [51].

Understanding CSCs is not only changing how scientists view cancer but also how they develop new strategies to prevent its return.

> ***A Patient's Perspective:*** Nora was a 39-year-old mother of two when she was diagnosed with an aggressive type of breast cancer. She underwent surgery, chemotherapy, and radiation. For a while, the scans were clear. But a year later, the cancer returned.
>
> Doctors told her that a small group of treatment-resistant cells may have survived the first round of therapy—possibly cancer stem cells. *"It was*

> *devastating," she said, "but also helped me understand that cancer isn't just about removing a lump—it's about targeting what caused it in the first place."*

Nora is now participating in a clinical trial testing a new drug designed to target cancer stem cells. Her story is a reminder that cancer is not always what it seems on the surface—and that new science is helping shape more effective treatments.

3.3 Similarities Between Stem Cells and Cancer Cells

At a cellular level, stem cells and cancer cells can sometimes exhibit remarkably similar behaviors. This has led researchers to study both types side by side, looking for clues that might help fight cancer.

Shared traits between stem cells and cancer stem cells:

- **Frequent Division**: Both stem cells and cancer cells can divide and multiply rapidly; however, in stem cells, this process is tightly regulated, whereas cancer cells grow uncontrollably.
- **Survival in Low-Oxygen (Hypoxic) Conditions**: Stem cells can thrive in low-oxygen niches in the body, which helps preserve them. Similarly, cancer cells often survive and even flourish in the low-oxygen areas of tumors [52].
- **Mobility**: During normal development, stem cells move to different parts of the body to form organs. Cancer cells hijack this ability during metastasis, allowing them to spread from the primary tumor to distant tissues [44].
- **Immune Evasion**: Normally, stem cells employ a clever survival strategy: they can **evade being attacked by the immune system**. This ability is essential because when the body is repairing itself—for example, after an injury—stem cells need time and protection to do their job without being mistakenly destroyed by the immune system's "soldiers."

  Unfortunately, cancer cells can **also employ this same tactic.** By disguising themselves or "turning off" the alarms that would usually alert the immune system, they manage to **slip under the radar**. Instead of being destroyed, these cancer cells are left alone to keep growing and spreading [53].

  This process, called **immune evasion**, is one of the reasons cancer can be so challenging to treat. It's also why modern research is focused on **immunotherapies** and stem-cell-based strategies that "unmask" cancer cells—making them visible again to the immune system so they can be destroyed.

Helpful Analogy

Think of the immune system as a city's **security force**, always on the lookout for intruders. Stem cells carry a special **"ID badge"** that tells the guards, "I belong here—don't attack me." Cancer cells, however, forge fake IDs or sneak past the cameras, pretending to be harmless. Because of this disguise, the guards overlook the intruders until it's too late.

These similarities are not just curiosities—they're key to understanding cancer. If cancer cells are using the same biological tricks as stem cells, researchers can use what they know about healthy stem cells to figure out what makes cancer so hard to treat.

But it's also crucial to identify the differences. Unlike normal stem cells, cancer cells do not follow the body's rules. They are selfish, relentless, and destructive. Scientists are now searching for molecular markers that separate the two cell types. These markers could become targets for precision therapies that disable cancer cells without harming the body's standard repair systems.

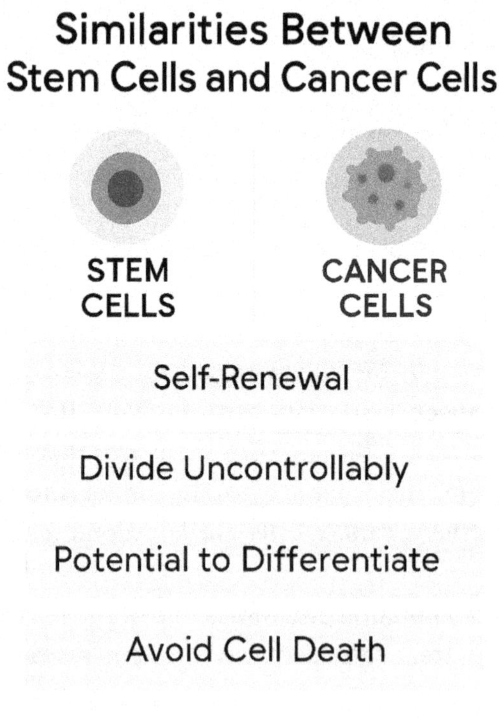

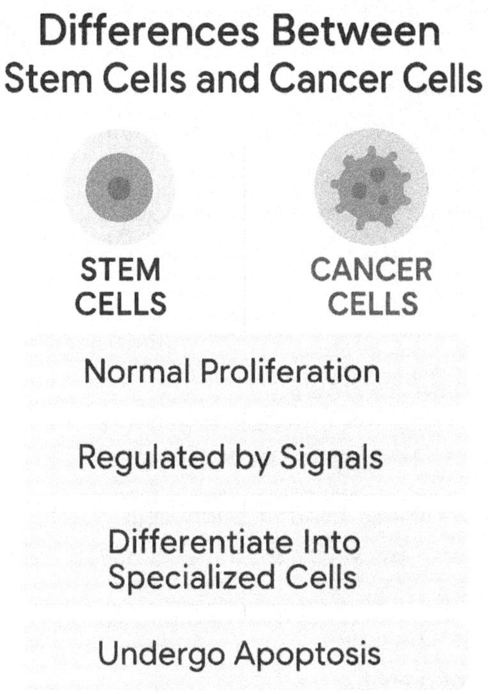

Understanding these parallels is helping researchers unravel one of cancer's deepest secrets—and offering new hope for smarter, more effective treatments.

3.4 Why Cancer Stem Cells Matter in Treatment

Most conventional cancer therapies—like chemotherapy and radiation—target fast-dividing tumor cells. While this can significantly reduce the visible tumor mass, it often leaves behind a small population of CSCs. These cells are often slow-dividing, resistant to standard treatments, and capable of initiating new tumors.

As a result:

- **Tumors may shrink but later return**, due to surviving CSCs that repopulate the tumor.
- **Metastasis may occur after seemingly successful treatment**, because CSCs can travel through the body and establish new tumors elsewhere.
- **Some cancers become harder to treat over time**, as CSCs evolve and become even more treatment-resistant.

New and emerging therapies are now being explicitly designed to target CSCs. These include:

- **Signal inhibitors**, which block cell molecular pathways such as Wnt, Notch, and Hedgehog, are critical for the survival of CSCs [54].
- **Immunotherapies** involve training or modifying the immune system to recognize and eliminate CSCs.
- **Combination therapies**, pairing conventional treatments with CSC-targeting drugs, are used to eradicate both the bulk tumor and its roots.

Targeting CSCs represents a critical advancement in the quest for more durable and effective cancer treatments, potentially preventing relapse and improving long-term survival rates.

3.5 Stem Cells as a Tool in Cancer Research

Researchers are also using healthy stem cells in the lab to model the formation of cancers. By watching how stem cells become abnormal, scientists can study:

- What genes trigger cancer
- How cancers respond to drugs
- How to prevent healthy stem cells from becoming cancerous

This has led to the development of **organoids**—miniature lab-grown organs made from stem cells. These tiny models allow researchers to test drugs in a way that mimics the human body without risking harm to patients [55].

3.6 The Future: Using Stem Cells to Fight Cancer

The future of cancer treatment may be closely tied to stem cells. Researchers around the world are exploring ways to use these versatile cells not only to fight cancer, but also to repair the damage it causes — as well as the damage caused by harsh treatments like chemotherapy and radiation. Below are some of the most promising approaches currently under investigation:

1. Regrowing tissue damaged by cancer or chemotherapy

Treatments like chemotherapy and radiation can effectively kill cancer cells, but they also harm healthy tissues, especially the bone marrow — the factory that produces blood. This damage often leads to **bone marrow suppression**, weakening the immune system and making recovery more difficult.

Hematopoietic stem cells (found in bone marrow and umbilical cord blood) are already used in transplants to **restore blood cell production** after high-dose cancer treatment – especially for leukemias and lymphomas. Scientists are now working to make this process **safer, more efficient, and applicable to a broader range of cancer types** [56].

2. Delivering anti-cancer drugs directly to tumors

One of the most exciting innovations in development is using stem cells as **"smart delivery vehicles."** Certain types of stem cells, like mesenchymal stem cells (MSCs), naturally migrate to areas of inflammation or tumors. Researchers are studying how to genetically modify these cells to carry cancer-fighting drugs or genes directly to the tumor – acting like a **"Trojan horse" against cancer** [57, 58].

This targeted approach could reduce the side effects of traditional chemotherapy by focusing the action directly on the cancer cells.

3. Boosting the immune system

Cell-based therapies are being combined with advances in immunotherapy. One promising idea is using stem cells to **generate specialized immune cells** that can more effectively recognize and target cancer cells. Scientists are exploring how to transform stem cells into customized **T cells, natural killer (NK) cells**, or **dendritic cells** – trained to fight cancer more precisely and effectively [59].

This approach has become increasingly popular and is being used in many cancer treatment centers.

4. Creating lab-grown tumor models for better drug testing

Induced pluripotent stem cells (iPSCs), which are adult cells reprogrammed to behave like embryonic stem cells, can be used to grow miniature organs or tumors – known as **organoids**.

These lab-grown models allow researchers to study how tumors develop and respond to treatments **without putting patients at risk**. This approach may accelerate the discovery of personalized cancer treatments and enhance outcomes [60].

5. Fixing cancer-causing genetic mutations

Looking to the future, scientists hope to combine stem cells with powerful tools that can "**edit**" **DNA** – like a high-precision pair of genetic scissors called **CRISPR-Cas9**. This would allow doctors to fix harmful changes (mutations) in a person's genes that can lead to cancer, especially in families where cancer runs in the genes.

Think of it like repairing a typo in your body's instruction manual before it causes a serious problem. In the future, doctors may be able to extract a person's cells, correct the cancer-related mutation in the lab, and then reintroduce the corrected cells to the body — potentially preventing cancer from developing altogether.

While this concept is still in early research stages, it opens the door to **personalized cancer prevention** [61, 62].

3.7 What's still needed?

Stem cell research in cancer therapy is one of the most promising areas in modern medicine—but it's still a work in progress. While some stem cell treatments (like bone marrow transplants) are already standard care, **many of the newer approaches are still in the laboratory or early clinical trials.** Scientists are proceeding with caution because the same powerful abilities that make stem cells useful can also create risks if not carefully controlled.

Some of the **significant challenges** include:

- **Preventing stem cells from turning cancerous themselves.**
  Since stem cells can grow and divide so effectively, there's always a small risk they might start dividing uncontrollably, just like cancer cells. Researchers are developing methods to closely monitor and regulate stem cell behavior to prevent this from happening.
- **Ensuring they behave as expected inside the body.**
  In the lab, scientists can guide stem cells to act in specific ways. But once they are returned to the body, the environment is more complex. Stem cells may migrate to unexpected locations or behave differently than anticipated. Understanding and predicting this behavior is crucial to ensuring the safety of treatments.
- **Making treatments safe, affordable, and accessible.**
  Even when therapies are effective, they must be tested in large patient groups to ensure long-term safety. Additionally, developing advanced stem cell treatments can be costly. Scientists, doctors, and policymakers are collaborating to find ways to reduce costs, ensuring these therapies are accessible to a broader range of people.

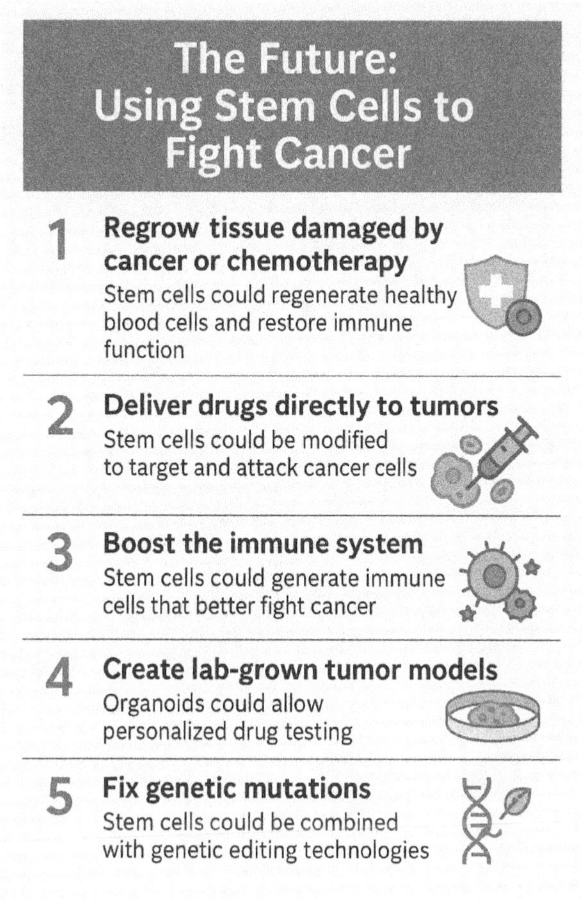

Despite these challenges, the outlook is **highly optimistic**. Advances in **biotechnology, bioengineering, and personalized medicine** are providing researchers with new tools to address these challenges—such as gene-editing systems to fine-tune stem cells or bioengineered "safety switches" that enable doctors to shut off stem cells if something goes wrong.

The field is evolving rapidly, and what is experimental today may soon become a **standard part of cancer care**. In the near future, stem cells could help usher in a new era of treatment that is not only more effective in fighting cancer but also gentler on patients, longer-lasting, **and personalized to each individual's needs.**

Helpful Analogy

Think of stem cell therapies like designing a **new type of airplane**. Engineers first test small models, then flight simulators, then carefully controlled test flights—making sure everything is safe before passengers ever board. In the same way, scientists must test stem cells step by step, solving challenges along the way, before these therapies become a part of everyday medicine.

Part II: The Science Behind the Therapy

Chapter 4 – Hematopoietic Stem Cells (HSCs) in Cancer Therapy

Hematopoietic stem cells (HSCs) are the "seed cells" that continuously replenish our blood and immune system. Hidden deep within the **bone marrow**, these extraordinary cells have the power to rebuild life from scratch—cell by cell.

In the context of cancer, HSCs have transformed from a biological curiosity into one of the most critical life-saving tools in modern medicine. For patients facing blood cancers like **leukemia, lymphoma,** or **multiple myeloma**, HSC transplantation can mean the difference between life and death. And with new scientific advances, their potential is expanding faster than ever before.

> ***Patient Quote:*** *"I was scared when my doctor said I needed a bone marrow transplant. But knowing it was stem cells rebuilding my blood and immune system gave me hope that my body could heal itself."* — Leah, 29.

4.1 The Basics: What Makes HSCs Special?

Most cells in our body have a single job—they might carry oxygen, send nerve signals, or produce hormones—but HSCs are multi-talented. They can **self-renew** (make identical copies of themselves) and **differentiate** (become any blood cell).

HSCs produce three prominent blood cell families:

1. Red blood cells (RBCs): Carry oxygen to tissues.

2. White blood cells (WBCs): Defend against infections.
3. **Platelets:** Help the blood clot to stop bleeding.

Every day, **your bone marrow produces billions of new blood cells**, and it is HSCs that sustain this process for decades.

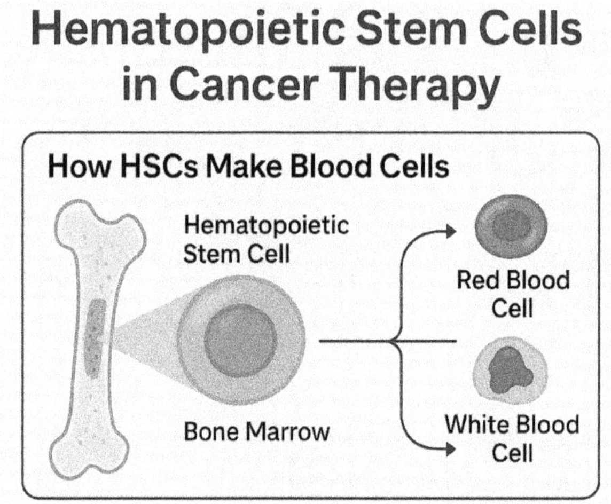

Key Points

- Hematopoietic stem cells (HSCs) are responsible for producing all types of blood cells.
- HSCs are primarily found in the bone marrow, the spongy tissue inside bones. HSCs are also found in cord blood.
- They can self-renew and differentiate into various types of blood cells, including red blood cells, white blood cells, and platelets.
- HSC transplants can be used in the treatment of some cancers and blood disorders.

4.2 Why Are HSCs Important in Cancer Therapy?

HSCs are often described as the lifeline of our blood and immune system. They live primarily in our bone marrow and have an incredible job: producing all the different types of blood cells we need to survive—oxygen-carrying red blood cells, infection-fighting white blood cells, and platelets that form clots. HSCs are found in bone marrow and cord blood. Every day, your body makes billions of new blood cells, and HSCs are the master builders behind this process.

A Key Ally in the Fight Against Cancer

In cancer therapy—especially for blood cancers like **leukemia, lymphoma,** and **multiple myeloma**, and even in **solid cancers like the breast**—HSCs can be life-saving. High-dose chemotherapy or radiation is often needed to destroy cancer cells. Still, these treatments also damage the patient's bone marrow, destroying the healthy cells needed to produce new blood.

This is where HSCs step in: by **rebuilding the blood and immune system** after aggressive treatment, they give patients a second chance at life. In many cases, HSC transplantation (often called a *bone marrow transplant*) is the only potential cure.

Why Doctors and Researchers Are Excited

Recent medical advances have made HSC therapy safer and more widely available than ever before:

- **Better donor matching** through global stem cell registries has dramatically improved transplant success rates [63].
- **Reduced-intensity conditioning** allows older patients and those with other health issues to benefit from transplants with fewer side effects [64].
- **Cord blood banking** has expanded the pool of potential donors, particularly for individuals from ethnic backgrounds that are underrepresented in donor registries [65].
- **Gene editing technologies** like CRISPR are showing potential to correct genetic defects in a patient's own HSCs before transplant—offering hope not just for cancer but for many inherited blood disorders [66].

Key Points

More than **50,000 stem cell transplants** are performed each year worldwide.

A Story of Renewal

Many patients often describe undergoing an HSC transplant as a chance to be *reborn*. Though the journey can be challenging, the outcomes are frequently remarkable. For example, an extensive study of patients with acute myeloid leukemia (AML) undergoing allogeneic stem cell transplantation found that approximately **19% remained disease-free at 10 years**, even in high-risk, hard-to-treat cases, demonstrating that long-term remission and cure are increasingly within reach [67].

This is not just about survival—it's about restoration. HSC therapy can restore immune function, reduce the risk of infection, and help patients return to their everyday lives. For a child with leukemia, it might mean going back to school; for an adult, it might mean returning to work, raising a family, or simply living without constant hospital visits.

Looking Ahead

The future is bright. Researchers are working on:

- **"Universal" donor cells** that could be given to any patient without risk of rejection.
- **Faster engraftment techniques** enable the immune system to recover in days instead of weeks.
- **Combination therapies** pairing HSC transplants with targeted cancer treatments for even better results.

Each year, thousands more lives are saved thanks to HSC therapy, and ongoing research promises to make it an even more powerful and accessible weapon against cancer.

4.3 Types of Hematopoietic Stem Cell (HSC) Transplants

HSC transplants are not a "one-size-fits-all" approach—there are different types, each chosen based on the patient's disease, health, and treatment goals. Think of them like different "delivery systems" for giving the body the fresh, healthy blood-making cells it needs.

1. Autologous Transplant – "Your Own Stem Cells, Back Again"

In this method, doctors collect the patient's **own** hematopoietic stem cells before high-dose chemotherapy or radiation. These healthy cells are carefully frozen and stored. After the cancer-killing treatment is completed, the stem cells are thawed and returned to the patient through an infusion, similar to a regular blood transfusion.

✓ **Best suited for:** Certain types of lymphomas and multiple myeloma.

✓ **Advantages:** No risk of immune rejection, because the cells are from the patient's own body.

‣ **Optimistic note:** Many patients report faster recovery times since the immune system recognizes its cells.

Analogy
Imagine removing precious seeds from a garden before a storm, keeping them safe, and then replanting them afterward to help the garden grow again.

2. Allogeneic Transplant – "A Donor's Gift"

In an allogeneic transplant, the stem cells come from a **donor**—often a closely matched sibling, another family member, or an unrelated volunteer from a donor registry.

✓**Best for:** Aggressive leukemias, some lymphomas, and inherited blood disorders.

✓**Advantages:** The donor's immune cells can launch what's called a **graft-versus-leukemia (GVL) effect**—essentially acting like an extra security team to track down and destroy any remaining cancer cells.

‣ **Optimistic note:** Donor transplants can offer an actual "fresh start," replacing the faulty blood system with one that's cancer-free. With better donor matching technology and improved immune system management, the risks are steadily going down.

> *Analogy*
> It's like bringing in a new, elite gardening crew to replace diseased plants and prevent weeds (cancer cells) from returning.

3. Cord Blood Transplant – "Stem Cells from New Beginnings"

Umbilical cord blood—collected after a healthy birth and stored in special cord banks—is a rich source of young, adaptable hematopoietic stem cells.

✓**Advantages:** Easier to find a match compared to traditional donors, and lower risk of severe graft-versus-host disease (GVHD).

‣ **Optimistic note:** These newborn cells are "naïve" and flexible, which can help them adapt better to the patient's body. Cord blood transplants have been vital for patients who can't find a matched donor quickly.

> *Analogy*
> Cord blood cells are like fresh, wild seeds that can grow in different types of soil, making them ideal when the perfect gardening conditions aren't available.

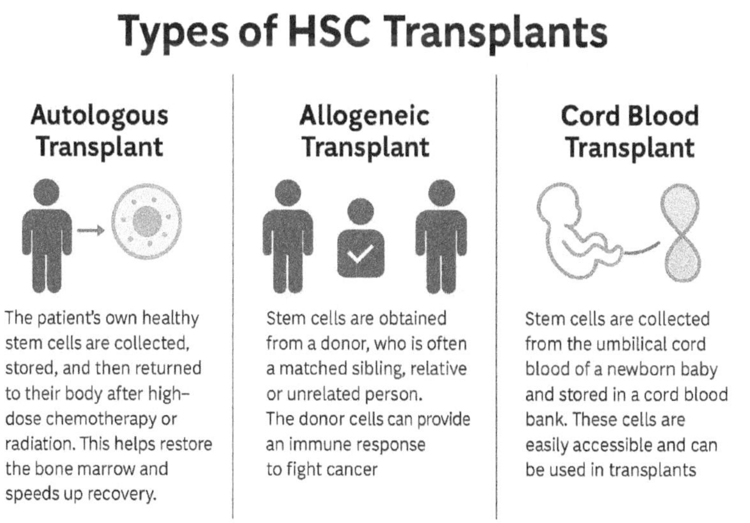

4.4 The Transplant Process (Step-by-Step)

Hematopoietic stem cell (HSC) transplantation might sound like a complex, high-tech procedure—and it is—but when broken down into steps, it's easier to understand. Think of it as a carefully orchestrated "reset" for the blood and immune system. Here's how the process works from start to finish:

1. Finding a Match

Doctors begin by looking for a donor whose immune system is closely compatible with the patient's. This is done through **HLA (human leukocyte antigen) typing,** a type of test that checks specific markers on white blood cells. A close match reduces the chance of the body rejecting the transplant.

- **Optimistic note:** Thanks to global donor registries, such as the National Marrow Donor Program and Bone Marrow Donors Worldwide, millions of potential donors are now searchable, meaning more patients find matches than ever before [63, 68].

2. Conditioning Treatment

Before the transplant, the patient undergoes **conditioning**, which usually involves high doses of chemotherapy, sometimes combined with radiation therapy. This step serves two purposes:

✓Destroy any remaining cancer cells.

✓Clear space in the bone marrow so the new stem cells can settle in and grow.

In some cases—especially for older patients or those with health concerns —**reduced-intensity conditioning** (a gentler approach) is used, making transplants possible for people who wouldn't have been eligible years ago [69].

3. Stem Cell Infusion

This is the moment when the transplant actually takes place. The donor's hematopoietic stem cells—collected from bone marrow, peripheral blood, or umbilical cord blood—are given to the patient **through a simple intravenous drip**, much like a regular blood transfusion. There's no surgery involved.

- **Optimistic note:** It's quick and painless, and many patients are surprised at how straightforward the "big day" feels.

4. Engraftment

Once infused, the stem cells travel through the bloodstream to the bone marrow, where they begin to "set up shop" and start producing healthy new blood cells. This process is called **engraftment** and usually takes **2–4 weeks.**

Signs of success include rising white blood cell counts, better immunity, and improved energy. Supportive care—such as antibiotics and growth factors—helps protect and accelerate recovery during this time.

5. Recovery

While engraftment is the first milestone, **complete immune system rebuilding can take months to years.** During this time, patients take extra precautions to avoid infections—such as wearing masks, washing their hands frequently, and avoiding crowds.

- **Optimistic note:** Advances in supportive medicine, antiviral therapies, and early warning systems for infections mean that transplant recovery is safer than ever before.

Many patients go on to live cancer-free, healthy lives, with some even returning to work, sports, and travel within a year.

4.5 Recent Advances Bringing Hope

In the past, hematopoietic stem cell transplants (HSCTs) were considered risky procedures that only the youngest and strongest patients could endure. Today, advances in science and medicine are transforming them into safer, more effective, and more widely accessible treatments—offering renewed hope for people with cancers like leukemia, lymphoma, and multiple myeloma.

Gentler, Safer Preparations – Reduced-Intensity Conditioning

Traditionally, HSCTs required very high doses of chemotherapy and radiation to destroy diseased bone marrow before the transplant. While effective, these regimens could be too toxic for older patients or those with other health conditions.

Now, reduced-intensity conditioning uses lower doses, making transplants safer while still allowing donor cells to take hold. This change has opened the door for patients in their 60s and even 70s to benefit from transplants [70, 71].

Better Matches, Better Outcomes – Improved Donor Matching

Finding a donor whose immune system closely matches that of the patient is critical for preventing complications such as graft-versus-host disease (GVHD). Thanks to **advanced genetic typing**, doctors can now match donors with unprecedented accuracy, even among unrelated volunteers. This precision has dramatically lowered the risk of complications and improved survival rates [72].

From Newborns to Adults – Cord Blood Expansion

Umbilical cord blood, rich in young stem cells, was once limited to treating children because it didn't contain enough cells for adults. However, **new laboratory techniques** now enable scientists to multiply these cells before transplant, making cord blood transplants a viable option for adults as well. This means that even patients without a matched donor can still receive life-saving treatment [73, 74].

Engineering Cells to Fight Back – Gene-Edited HSCs

One of the most exciting new frontiers in medicine is the use of **gene-editing tools**, such as **CRISPR-Cas9**, for the precise editing of human hematopoietic stem cells before they are returned to the patient. Think of it as giving these stem cells a tune-up in the lab. Scientists can "arm" them in different ways: sometimes by fixing a weakness that cancer could exploit, other times by adding new instructions that make the immune system stronger and more alert to cancer cells. The hope is that once these enhanced stem cells are back in the body, they can build an army of healthy, cancer-fighting blood and immune cells. This approach could not only reduce the risk of the cancer coming back (a relapse) but also, in the future, lead to long-term cures for certain types of cancer.[75, 76].

> *Analogy*
> Using CRISPR on stem cells is like upgrading a computer's software before reinstalling it. By fixing bugs and adding new features, the system operates more smoothly and can better defend itself against future problems.

The Results Are Showing

The impact of these innovations is already being seen. Recent studies have reported steadily improving 5-year survival rates, especially in younger patients and for aggressive blood cancers once considered untreatable [77, 78]. Every year, thousands more patients worldwide receive HSCTs safely—and live to see years they never thought they would have.

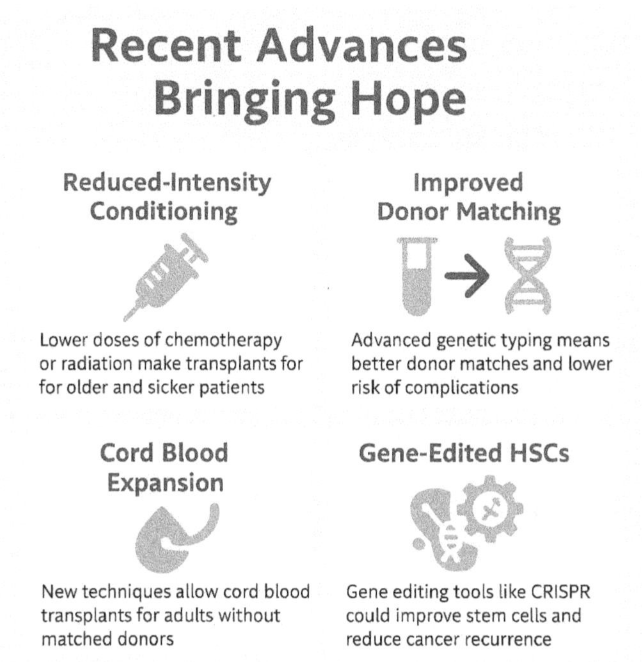

4.6 Understanding the Risks – and Why the Future Looks Brighter

HSC transplants offer a chance at life, especially for patients with blood cancers. However, the journey presents some significant challenges. Here's what can happen—and how modern science is making the path smoother:

1. Graft-Versus-Host Disease (GVHD)

What's the risk? When donor immune cells perceive the patient's body as "foreign," they can attack healthy tissues, including the skin, gut, liver, and more. This is known as GVHD and can be either acute or chronic.

How we are combating it positively:

✓ **Post-transplant cyclophosphamide (PTCy):** A safer method involving giving low-dose chemotherapy after infusion has dramatically lowered GVHD rates, even with partial donor matches (haploidentical transplants), expanding the pool of donors for many patients [79, 80]

✓**New medications for chronic GVHD:** Recently approved oral treatments, such as **ibrutinib**, **ruxolitinib**, and **belumosudil**, offer effective relief when standard treatments fail, with better outcomes and fewer side effects [81].

These advances mean that GVHD is no longer a deal-breaker, even for patients without a perfect donor.

2. Risk of Infection and Immunodeficiency

Because HSC transplants temporarily suppress the immune system, infections pose a significant threat during recovery.

Hopeful progress includes:

✓**Vaccination strategies:** Patients restart essential vaccines—such as influenza, pneumonia, and COVID-19—as early as three months post-transplant, following structured guidelines designed to build protection safely [82].

✓**Monitoring vaccine response:** Studies show that up to 86% of patients develop protective immunity from COVID-19 vaccines, especially when receiving three or more doses—highlighting that vaccines are both safe and effective in HSC recipients [83].

These efforts are helping to restore patient immunity more quickly, thereby protecting against serious, preventable infections.

3. Infections in Chronic GVHD

Long-term GVHD and its treatments often leave patients especially vulnerable to infections.

✓**Tailored prevention strategies:** Healthcare teams now adapt infection monitoring and treatment based on each patient's specific immune profile, significantly reducing risks [84, 85].

Challenge	Positive Breakthroughs
GVHD	More effective prevention strategies and new treatments
Infections	Faster immunity through safe vaccination protocols
Long-term care	Personalized monitoring to prevent lingering complications

Why This Brings Real Hope

Instead of presenting barriers, these improvements are turning HSC transplantation into safer, more manageable, and increasingly accessible treatment—bringing renewed health back to life for thousands of patients each year.

4.7 The Future: Beyond Today's Limits

The future of **hematopoietic stem cell (HSC) therapy** is brighter than ever. What once seemed like science fiction—using stem cells to reset or even redesign the body's immune system—is now becoming a real possibility.

Researchers are working on innovations that could make these therapies not only safer and faster but also accessible to more people around the world.

Universal Donor Cells

One of the biggest obstacles in stem cell transplantation is finding the right **donor match**. Just like with organ transplants, the immune system is very particular—it looks for tiny genetic "ID tags" on cells, known as **tissue types.** If the donor's tissue type doesn't closely match the patient's, the new cells may be seen as intruders. This can trigger a serious complication such as GVHD, where the transplanted cells begin attacking the patient's body.

Today, patients sometimes wait months—or even years—for a suitable donor. This delay can be dangerous, especially for people with aggressive cancers who need treatment quickly.

To solve this problem, scientists are working on creating **"universal donor" hematopoietic stem cells (HSCs)**. These are specially engineered stem cells designed to be accepted by any patient, regardless of their genetic background. In other words, they would act like a **universal blood type**—safe to give to anyone [86-89]. If this technology succeeds, it could **transform cancer care**. Patients would no longer need to wait anxiously for a donor match, and doctors could provide **life-saving transplants immediately**. It would also make treatments more equitable, ensuring access for patients in countries or communities where donor registries are limited.

Researchers are still testing how to make these universal cells both **effective and safe**, but early progress is promising. The vision is clear: a future where every patient who needs a stem cell transplant can receive one —without waiting, without searching, and without the same risk of life-threatening complications.

This would mean no more waiting for a donor match, dramatically speeding up life-saving treatments.

> *Analogy*
> Think of donor cells like **keys** and the patient's immune system like a **lock**. Usually, only one specific key will fit a lock, so doctors must search for the perfect match. But universal donor stem cells are like a **master key**—they're designed to open any lock safely. With a master key, there's no more searching, no more waiting—just a direct solution when it's needed most.

"Designer Immunity" Against Cancer

Imagine if stem cells could be programmed like software to create an immune system that actively hunts down and destroys cancer. Advances in genetic engineering and CRISPR technology are bringing this dream closer to reality. Researchers are learning how to **reprogram HSCs to generate supercharged immune cells**, such as natural killer (NK) cells or T cells, that can recognize and wipe out cancer cells more effectively than before [90, 91].

Combining HSC Therapy with CAR-T Cells

CAR-T cell therapy, where a patient's own T cells are engineered to fight cancer, has already changed the lives of many people with blood cancers. Now, researchers are exploring ways to **combine CAR-T therapy with HSC transplants**. The goal is to provide patients not only with an army of cancer-fighting immune cells but also with a long-lasting, healthy blood and immune system to sustain remission. Early clinical trials suggest this combination may offer more durable cures, especially in aggressive leukemias and lymphomas [90, 92, 93].

Faster, Safer, and More Widely Available

New techniques are being developed to shorten recovery times, reduce the risk of infections, and minimize side effects. For example, some studies are using **ex vivo expanded HSCs** (cells grown and multiplied in the lab before transplant) to speed bone marrow recovery. Others are exploring **off-the-shelf stem cell products**, meaning hospitals could have ready-to-use cells available without delay [94-98].

Experts predict that within the next decade, **HSC therapy will not only be more effective but also widely available outside of major cancer centers,** bringing hope to patients in smaller hospitals and even in developing regions. The vision is that one day, stem cell therapy may become as routine as chemotherapy is today—but with fewer side effects and more lasting benefits.

In simple terms
The future of HSC therapy isn't just about treating cancer—it's about **transforming the way we heal,** offering people not just survival but a return to whole, healthy, and vibrant lives.

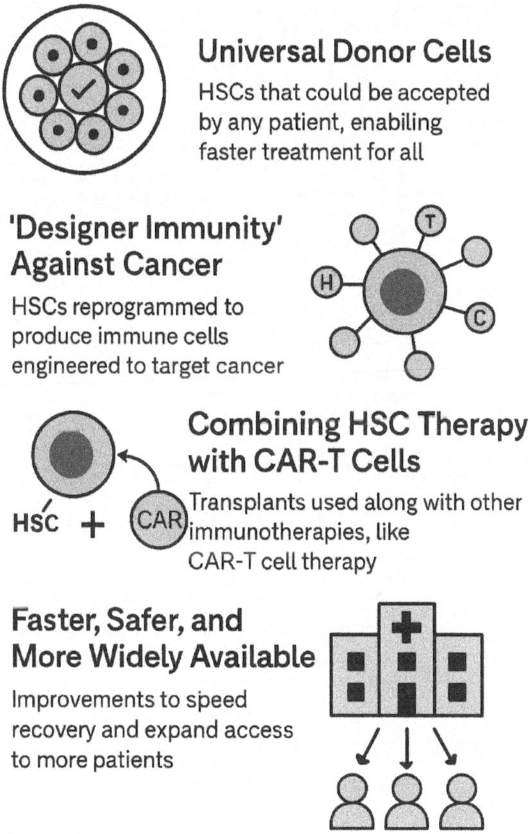

Chapter 5 – Mesenchymal Stem Cells in Cancer Research and Treatment

Mesenchymal stem cells, or MSCs, are among the most extensively studied types of stem cells in contemporary medical research. These remarkable cells can be found in the bone marrow, fat tissue, umbilical cord tissue, dental pulp, and even the uterine lining. Their unique ability to become bone, fat, or cartilage cells, along with their powerful healing and anti-inflammatory properties, makes them promising candidates for treating a wide range of diseases—including cancer.

But their role in cancer is complex. While some studies suggest MSCs can help fight cancer, others show they might unintentionally support tumor growth. In this chapter, we'll explore how MSCs work, what makes them valuable in cancer research, and the challenges scientists are working to overcome.

> ***Patient Quote:*** *"When I joined a trial using MSCs to help with side effects, it felt like being part of something bigger—not just for me, but for future patients too."* — James, 58.

5.1 What Are Mesenchymal Stem Cells?

MSCs are a type of adult stem cell, meaning they are found in fully developed tissues and play a crucial role in repair and maintenance throughout life. Unlike embryonic stem cells, MSCs do not carry the same ethical concerns and can be collected from a patient's own body (autologous source) or a donor (allogeneic source). They are present in multiple tissues—including bone marrow, adipose tissue (fat), umbilical cord tissue, dental pulp, and even the synovial membrane of joints.

From a biological standpoint, MSCs are prized for their versatility. They have several defining characteristics:

- **Multipotency** – The ability to transform into multiple types of specialized cells, most notably bone cells (osteocytes), cartilage cells (chondrocytes), and fat cells (adipocytes). This adaptability is central to their regenerative potential.
- **Tissue repair** – MSCs act like a cellular repair crew, migrating to areas of injury or inflammation and releasing biological proteins known as growth factors that stimulate healing.
- **Immunomodulation** – MSCs can fine-tune immune system activity, reducing excessive inflammation, which is valuable in treating autoimmune diseases and preventing transplant rejection.
- **Homing ability** – Guided by chemical signals released from damaged or diseased tissues, MSCs can locate and move toward sites of injury, chronic inflammation, or tumors.

Their combined abilities make MSCs promising candidates for therapies targeting not only orthopedic conditions like osteoarthritis but also cardiovascular diseases, neurodegenerative disorders such as Parkinson's and Alzheimer's, and various forms of cancer [14, 99].

Delivering Anti-Cancer Agents

Because MSCs naturally home to tumors, scientists have begun engineering them to carry anti-cancer agents—such as chemotherapy drugs, immune-activating molecules, or even oncolytic viruses (viruses designed to infect and kill cancer cells specifically). This targeted delivery approach can concentrate the treatment at the tumor site, reducing harm to healthy tissues and potentially lowering side effects [100, 101]. In laboratory and early animal studies, MSCs loaded with such agents have successfully slowed tumor growth and limited metastasis.

Modifying the Tumor Microenvironment

The biological environment surrounding a tumor, known as the **tumor microenvironment,** comprises blood vessels, immune cells, connective tissue, and various signaling molecules. It plays a significant role in how tumors grow and spread [102]. MSCs can be used to deliver substances that disrupt this environment, making it harder for cancer to thrive. For example, they may be modified to release molecules that stop new blood vessels from forming (anti-angiogenic factors), starving the tumor of nutrients and oxygen [103, 104]. This approach aims to weaken the tumor's support system from the inside.

Immune System Enhancement

Researchers are exploring ways to reprogram MSCs so that, when they arrive at a tumor site, they release cytokines—proteins that alert and activate immune cells. This can boost the body's natural ability to recognize and destroy cancer cells. Some experimental designs combine MSC delivery with immune checkpoint inhibitors, creating a double attack that both exposes and kills hidden tumor cells.

Reducing Side Effects of Cancer Treatments

Beyond attacking tumors, MSCs are also being studied for their ability to protect and heal healthy tissues during cancer treatment. Because they release anti-inflammatory factors and support tissue regeneration, MSCs may help reduce gut inflammation caused by radiation therapy, speed the repair of damaged skin, and restore bone marrow function after chemotherapy. In some trials, patients who received MSCs after undergoing bone marrow transplants recovered their immune function more quickly and experienced fewer complications.

Overall, each of these strategies is still under careful study. Still, together they highlight the versatility of MSCs as both a weapon against cancer and a shield for the patient's healthy cells [105, 106].

> 💡 ***Did You Know?***
> MSCs act like the body's natural **"repair crew."**

5.2 The Double-Edged Sword: MSCs and Tumor Promotion

Despite their potential, MSCs are not without risks. Some studies suggest MSCs may unintentionally support tumor growth by:

- Suppressing the immune system too much.
- Promoting blood vessel formation (angiogenesis), which feeds tumors.
- Encouraging the spread (metastasis) of certain types of cancer.

These effects depend on several factors, including the type of cancer, the source of the MSCs, the method of modification, and the mode of administration. It is one reason why MSC-based therapies for cancer are still largely experimental and are being tested in carefully controlled clinical trials.

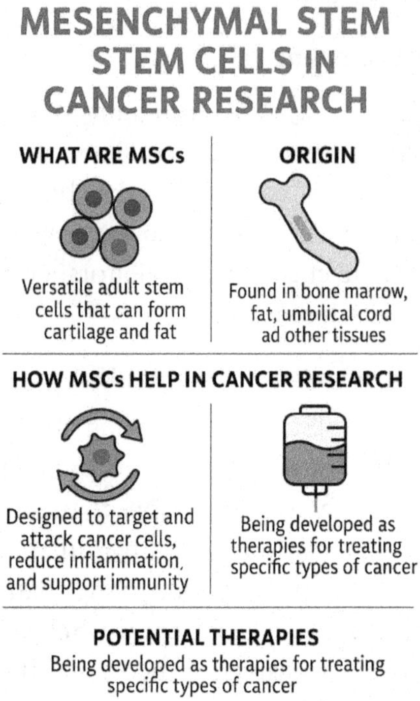

5.3 Clinical Trials and Current Studies

Many clinical trials worldwide are now investigating the safe and effective use of MSCs in cancer therapy. These trials encompass a range of strategies, from directly targeting tumors to supporting patient recovery after intensive treatments. For instance, some studies are focused on highly aggressive cancers like glioblastoma and metastatic melanoma, where MSCs are engineered to deliver potent anti-tumor agents. Others explore their use in more common cancers such as breast and prostate cancer, aiming to prevent recurrence or slow disease progression. In blood cancers like leukemia, MSCs are being tested for their ability to speed immune recovery after bone marrow transplantation.

Another primary focus is on supportive care, as trials investigate whether MSCs can reduce radiation-induced tissue damage, alleviate chemotherapy-related gut inflammation, and enhance overall patient quality of life during treatment.

As of 2024, over 200 trials involving MSCs and cancer have been registered on major databases such as ClinicalTrials.gov [107]. While most are still in early stages (Phase I or II), some have advanced to later phases, evaluating not just safety but also long-term effectiveness and survival outcomes [107]. Clinical trials cover a broad spectrum of cancers from aggressive brain tumors like glioblastoma to skin cancers such as metastatic melanoma, as well as common malignancies like breast and prostate cancer. Early findings are promising in terms of reduced side effects and improved recovery times; however, the results are mixed when it comes to directly shrinking tumors.

Researchers emphasize that MSC therapy is not a one-size-fits-all solution. The optimal source of MSCs, the method of modification, and the route of administration may vary significantly depending on the type and stage of cancer. These ongoing studies are crucial for determining which patients are most likely to benefit and for maximizing safety while preserving the therapeutic potential of MSCs.

5.4 A Patient's Perspective: Lucas' Journey

Lucas, a 10-year-old boy with relapsed leukemia, participated in an MSC trial designed to boost immune recovery after his bone marrow transplant. His *cancer journey* illustrates the human side of cutting-edge science. After enduring months of intense treatments, Lucas was physically drained and at high risk of infection. The trial offered something beyond medicine—it provided a path forward. His mother recalls:

> ***A Patient's Perspective:*** *"It was terrifying at first—we didn't know what to expect. However, the doctors explained how the stem cells might help him recover more quickly, strengthen his defenses, and improve his overall quality of life. Watching him regain his energy, smile again, and even play with his friends sooner than we imagined was nothing short of miraculous. It gave us hope, and for us, that hope made all the difference."*

5.5 The Path Forward

MSCs hold extraordinary promise as a versatile and potentially transformative tool in the fight against cancer. While careful study is still essential to ensure safety and effectiveness, each year brings new insights and breakthroughs. Researchers are advancing precision-targeting methods, decoding the complex interactions between MSCs and tumors, and tailoring therapies to match each patient's specific cancer type and stage. With every successful trial and refinement, the vision of safer, more personalized, and highly effective stem cell–based treatments moves closer to becoming a reality, offering renewed hope for patients and families worldwide.

> *Did You Know?*
> MSCs were first discovered in bone marrow, but are also in fat, skin, and dental pulp.

5.6 The Future of Stem Cell Therapies in Cancer Treatment

A New Era of Hope

For decades, cancer has been one of the toughest challenges in medicine. But today, thanks to stem cell research, we are entering a new era filled with hope. Scientists are no longer just focusing on killing cancer cells – they are also finding ways to *help the body heal itself.* MSCs, with their unique ability to regenerate, repair, and interact with other cells, play a central role in this transformation.

1. Smarter, Safer Stem Cells

Researchers are engineering stem cells to act like tiny "smart packages." These cells can carry powerful cancer-killing drugs, immune-boosting proteins, or even viruses designed to attack tumors – and deliver them **only** where they are needed. This could mean fewer side effects compared to traditional chemotherapy.

> ***Optimism***
> Imagine treatments that fight cancer without making patients lose their hair, damage their heart, or weaken their immune system. That's the vision driving much of today's work.

2. Repairing the Damage of Cancer Treatments

Chemotherapy and **radiation treatments** have saved countless lives by destroying cancer cells. As they are so powerful, they don't just target cancer–they can also hurt healthy tissues. This can leave behind lasting problems, such as **bone marrow suppression**, where the body struggles to produce enough blood cells, or **damage to organs** like the heart, lungs, or digestive system.

This is where stem cells may offer new hope. Scientists are testing them in clinical trials to see if they can help the body heal from these side effects. For example, **HSCs** are already used to help patients recover their blood counts and immunity after chemotherapy. Meanwhile, **MSCs** are being studied for their ability to act like the body's natural repair crew, with early studies showing they may help mend tissues injured by radiation, such as the skin, the lining of the intestines, and even the tiny salivary glands that keep the mouth moist.

The goal is not just to fight the cancer, but also to **restore quality of life** so that patients can heal more fully after treatment.

> ***Analogy***
> Think of chemotherapy and radiation like a storm that tears through a town—knocking down houses and damaging roads while clearing away dangerous weeds. Stem cells act like a team of **construction workers,** coming in afterward to repair what was broken, rebuild the foundations, and make the system strong again.

> ***Optimism***
> Future therapies may not only cure cancer but also leave survivors healthier and stronger than before.

3. Boosting the Immune System

One of the most exciting areas of research today is the combination of **stem cells** with **immunotherapy**—a type of treatment that helps the body's own immune system identify and destroy cancer cells. Typically, cancer cells are stealthy; they can disguise themselves to evade detection, much like criminals hiding from the police. Immunotherapy works by training immune cells, such as T cells, to recognize these "disguises" and attack the cancer.

Now, scientists are investigating how **engineered stem cells** may enhance this process even further. In early studies, stem cells have been modified in the laboratory to deliver signals or substances that "**teach**" **immune cells** how to identify cancer more effectively. This teamwork could help the immune system track down hidden cancer cells that would otherwise escape notice. By combining the natural healing power of stem cells with the targeted attack of immunotherapy, researchers aim to develop treatments that are both more effective and longer-lasting.

Analogy
Imagine the immune system as a **police force** patrolling the body. Cancer cells are like clever criminals in disguise, blending in to avoid capture. Immunotherapy acts as a detective, revealing to the immune system who the real criminals are. **Stem cells, when engineered in the lab, act like teachers at the police academy—giving officers new skills and sharper instincts to catch even the most hidden offenders.**

Optimism
This could mean fewer relapses and long-lasting remission, turning cancer into a disease that can be *controlled — or even eliminated permanently*.

4. Personalized Stem Cell Medicine

No two cancers are exactly alike—just as no two people are identical. Even when two patients have the same type of cancer, the genetic "fingerprints" of their tumors can be very different. This means a treatment that works well for one person may not be as effective for another.

That's why scientists are working on ways to create **personalized therapies** using a patient's own stem cells. The idea is to take stem cells from the patient—like drawing a sample of blood or bone marrow—then carefully engineer them in the lab to recognize and fight the unique mutations in that person's cancer. These engineered cells could then be returned to the patient, acting as a custom-made treatment tailored to match their disease.

Analogy
Think of personalized stem cell therapy like having a **tailor make a custom suit**. The tailor measures every detail of your body to create clothing made just for you. In the same way, doctors can use a person's own stem cells to design a therapy that "fits" the exact shape of their cancer, offering a treatment that is precise and personal.

Optimism
Instead of a "one-size-fits-all" treatment, future cancer care may be custom-tailored to each individual, offering the best chance of success with the fewest risks.

This approach is becoming increasingly realistic as advances in **genetics** and **cell engineering** enable doctors to map out the exact changes in a tumor's DNA and design targeted countermeasures. While still in the research stage, personalized stem cell therapy holds the promise of more effective treatments, causing fewer side effects, and providing each patient with a plan tailored to their own biology.

5.7 A Global Vision for the Next Decade

Currently, there are more than 400 clinical trials worldwide testing stem cell-based approaches for cancer. That number is growing every year, demonstrating the significant interest and momentum this field has garnered. Each trial, whether big or small, adds a valuable piece to the puzzle—helping scientists refine techniques, improve safety, and discover what works best for patients.

Of course, challenges remain. Doctors must ensure that these therapies are not only powerful but also **safe in the long term**. Meanwhile, researchers are working diligently to make treatments more affordable, enabling them to reach people everywhere. But the progress made so far is nothing short of remarkable—and it is accelerating faster than ever before.

The most exciting part is what lies ahead. Treatments that are considered **experimental today may become routine in the near future**. Within the next decade, stem cell therapies may become a standard part of cancer care, offering patients options that are **more effective, less toxic, and tailored to their individual needs**. For millions of people worldwide, this could mean not only better survival but also a better quality of life during and after treatment.
It's a future that feels closer every day—and one that offers real hope that science and compassion, working together, can transform the fight against cancer.

Optimism
The next generation may grow up in a world where MSC therapies are a standard part of cancer care, offering hope not just for survival but for *proper healing*.

Mesenchymal Stem Cells in Cancer Research

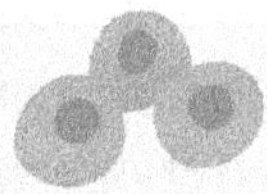

What They Are

Adult stem cells found in bone marrow and other tissues

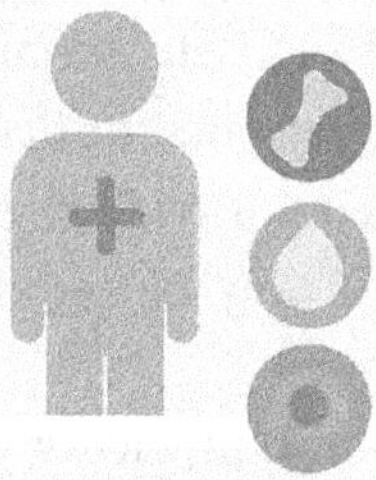

Roles in the Body

Help create bone, cartilage, fat, and more; modulate the immune system

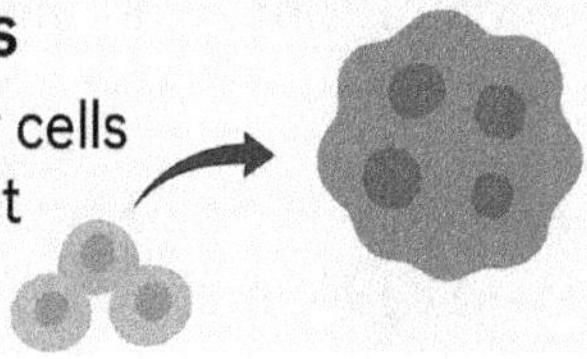

Targeting Tumors

Can seek out cancer cells and deliver treatment directly to tumors

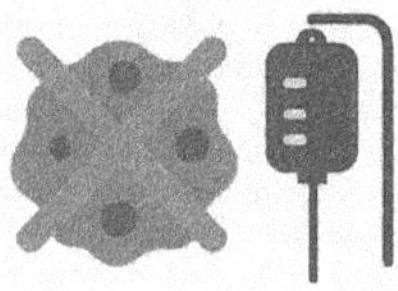

Suppressing Cancer

May inhibit tumor growth and support other therapies

Chapter 6 – How Stem Cells May Help Treat Cancer

Introduction

> ***A Patient's Perspective:*** When Sarah was diagnosed with an aggressive form of breast cancer at just 38 years old, she braced herself for the long road ahead—surgery, chemotherapy, radiation. She endured months of treatment, emerging exhausted but hopeful. Yet, the cancer returned two years later. Faced with limited options, Sarah enrolled in an early-stage clinical trial using her stem cells to deliver targeted cancer therapy. *"It felt like a leap into the unknown,"* she recalls. *"But it also felt like hope."*

Cancer is not an invader from the outside—it begins within us, in our cells. Under normal circumstances, our cells grow, divide, and die in an orderly fashion, much like a well-rehearsed symphony. But when this harmony is disrupted, specific cells begin to grow uncontrollably, ignore the body's natural "stop signals," and sometimes spread to other parts of the body. This uncontrolled growth can interfere with vital functions, weaken organs, and, if unchecked, become life-threatening.

Over the last century, medical science has made tremendous strides in cancer treatment. Surgery can remove solid tumors, chemotherapy can target rapidly dividing cells, and radiotherapy can destroy cancer with carefully focused beams of energy. These treatments have saved millions of lives and continue to improve in safety and effectiveness. Yet, they also have limitations: they can harm healthy tissues, cause severe side effects such as fatigue, nausea, and immune suppression, and in some cases, fail to eliminate every last cancer cell—allowing the disease to return.

HOW STEM CELLS MAY HELP TREAT CANCER

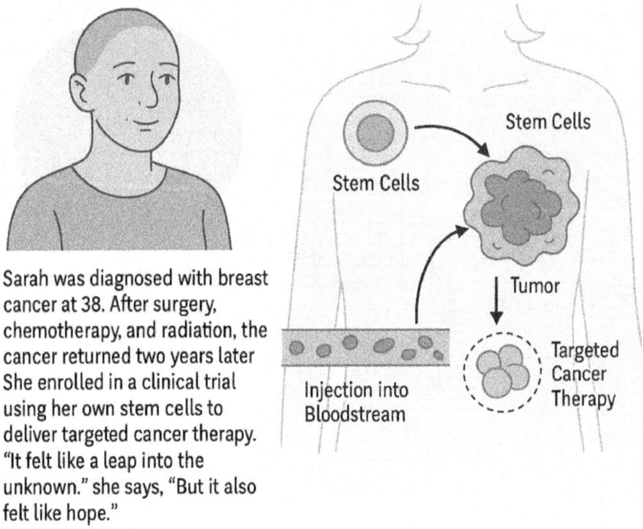

On the left, Sarah's story as a breast cancer patient is introduced with a simple, stylized portrait, conveying her journey through treatment and a clinical trial with stem cells to target her cancer, symbolizing hope. On the right, a clear diagram illustrates how stem cells are utilized in targeted cancer therapy, with arrows indicating the process of their injection and interaction with the tumor.

This is where **stem cell research** comes into play—a rapidly advancing field that offers new hope. Stem cells are unlike ordinary cells: they have the extraordinary ability to repair damaged tissues, regulate the immune system, and, in some cases, travel directly to sites of disease, including tumors. Scientists are now learning how to harness these natural abilities, not just to fight cancer more precisely, but to help the body recover and stay healthier after treatment.

Imagine a treatment that could seek out and destroy cancer cells without harming healthy ones... or help regrow tissues damaged by radiation... or boost the immune system so it remains vigilant against cancer's return. These ideas are no longer confined to science fiction—they are the focus of active research and early clinical trials happening around the world today.

In this chapter, we will examine how various types of stem cells may contribute to **the fight against cancer**. We'll break down the science into clear, understandable concepts, highlight promising research, and share real-world patient experiences. By the end, you'll see why many scientists believe stem cells could one day stand alongside surgery, chemotherapy, and radiotherapy as a powerful, life-saving tool in the battle against cancer.

> ***Patient Quote:*** *"Chemo saved my life, but it also left me exhausted and weak. Hearing that stem cells might one day repair this kind of damage made me feel hopeful for patients who come after me."* — Aisha, 41.

6.1 Understanding the Key Players: Types of Stem Cells in Cancer Treatment

Before diving into applications, it's essential to understand the main types of stem cells being explored:

1. **Mesenchymal Stem Cells (MSCs)** – Found in bone marrow, fat tissue, umbilical cord, and other sources. They are known for their **homing ability** (moving toward injury or tumor sites), **anti-inflammatory effects**, and capacity to differentiate into multiple cell types [14].
2. **Hematopoietic Stem Cells (HSCs)** – Found in bone marrow and blood. These are the stem cells responsible for making all blood cells. They are **already used clinically** in bone marrow transplants for blood cancers, such as leukemia and lymphoma [56].
3. **Induced Pluripotent Stem Cells (iPSCs)** – Laboratory-created stem cells generated from adult cells. **They can be programmed to become almost any type of cell.** In cancer research, iPSCs are being investigated for the production of personalized immune cells [21].

6.2 Using Stem Cells as Cancer-Fighting Delivery Vehicles

One of the most exciting and widely studied applications of stem cells in oncology is their use as **"living delivery vehicles"**—sometimes referred to as the **Trojan Horse strategy**. In this approach, scientists capitalize on the natural tendency of specific stem cells—particularly mesenchymal stem cells (MSCs)—to **migrate** to areas of tissue damage, inflammation, or tumor growth.

This tumor-seeking property means that stem cells can potentially be **loaded** or **engineered** to carry therapeutic agents directly to the cancer site, bypassing much of the healthy tissue and concentrating treatment where it is needed most.

How It Works

Tumors release a range of **chemical signals**, such as chemokines[3] (e.g., CXCL12) and growth factors (e.g., VEGF), which serve to attract cells that can help them grow and survive. MSCs respond to these signals through specific chemokine receptors[4] (such as CXCR4), enabling them to migrate toward the tumor microenvironment [108].

Once MSCs arrive at the tumor site, they can be **modified** or **preloaded** to release cancer-killing payloads, including:

- **Chemotherapy drugs** – Instead of flooding the whole body with chemotherapy—which can damage healthy tissues—scientists are learning how to program stem cells to travel directly to tumors. Once there, the stem cells can release their "payload" of cancer-fighting drugs exactly where they're needed most. This approach could make treatments both more effective and less toxic, thereby reducing side effects such as nausea, hair loss, and fatigue. MSCs can also be engineered to produce and secrete pro-drug–activating enzymes. These enzymes convert harmless compounds into active chemotherapy drugs directly inside the tumor [109].
- **Oncolytic viruses** – MSCs can be used as carriers for viruses that specifically infect and destroy cancer cells while leaving healthy cells untouched. This method also stimulates an immune response against the tumor [101, 110].
- **Immune-activating molecules (cytokines)** – MSCs can deliver signaling proteins, such as interferon-beta (IFN-β) or interleukin-12 (IL-12), which alert and activate nearby immune cells to attack the tumor [111].
- **Pro-apoptotic proteins** – These trigger programmed cell death in cancer cells, targeting them without harming normal cells [58].

Benefits of the Trojan Horse Approach

Compared to traditional cancer therapies, MSC-based delivery systems offer several potential advantages:

1. **Precision Targeting** – The treatment is concentrated in the tumor, sparing healthy tissues from exposure.

[3] Chemokines are small messenger proteins that act like "chemical GPS signals," guiding immune cells to where they're needed in the body.

[4] Chemokine receptors are tiny "antennae" on the surface of cells that detect chemokine signals and guide the cells to the right location.

2. **Reduced Side Effects** – Since healthy cells are spared mainly, systemic toxicity (such as nausea, hair loss, or immune suppression) can be significantly reduced.
3. **Access to Hidden Tumors** – MSCs can migrate into **deep-seated tumors** and even infiltrate metastatic sites that are hard to reach with surgery or drugs.
4. **Sustained Release** – Engineered stem cells can act as "mini factories," releasing therapeutic agents over an extended period rather than all at once.

Real-World and Preclinical Examples: Signs of a Brighter Future

Encouraging research from around the world shows that stem cell–based delivery systems are more than just a theory—they're already demonstrating remarkable results:

- **Allogeneic MSCs Engineered to Release Interferon-β (2024)**
  Researchers have created MSCs modified to both promote cancer cell death and regulate immune responses. These cells were designed to lack interferon receptor 1, allowing them to deliver interferon-β directly to tumors with enhanced safety and efficacy. The results show promising potential in boosting cancer cell elimination and immune support [111].
- **MSC-Derived Cytokine Delivery (2025)**
  Recent studies highlight MSCs' ability to act as effective "cytokine factories." For instance, MSCs engineered to express IL-2 significantly regressed glioma tumors and improved survival in experimental models. MSCs modified to secrete IFN-α exhibited strong anti-tumor effects in a multiple myeloma experimental model, demonstrating the power of localized cytokine delivery [112, 113].
- **Broad MSC Applications in Cancer Therapy (2024)**
  These cells have a natural ability to "home in" on tumors—almost like they have a built-in GPS that guides them to sites of disease. Scientists are harnessing this unique property as a powerful tool for combating cancer.

  Instead of relying solely on drugs that circulate throughout the entire body, MSCs can be used as delivery vehicles to bring treatments directly into the tumor's microenvironment. Once they arrive, they can release a variety of cancer-fighting agents, including:

  ✓ MicroRNAs: tiny molecules that can switch genes on or off, shutting down processes cancer cells need to grow.

✓Drugs: traditional chemotherapy medicines loaded into MSCs so they go straight to the tumor, reducing harm to healthy tissues.

✓Oncolytic viruses: special viruses engineered to infect and kill cancer cells without harming normal cells.

In 2024, reviews of the field highlight just how far this approach has come. Scientists are no longer only testing whether MSCs can carry therapies—they are actively engineering MSCs to make them more accurate, safer, and longer-lasting inside the body. For example, new genetic tweaks able MSCs to recognize cancer cells more precisely, while safety switches are being incorporated so that the cells can be turned off if needed.

The vision is clear: MSCs could become a versatile "toolbox" in cancer therapy, able to carry different kinds of weapons depending on the patient's cancer. What once seemed futuristic is now rapidly moving toward reality, with the hope that these engineered stem cells will provide doctors with new ways to target tumors while sparing healthy tissue [101].

Analogy

Think of MSCs as **delivery drones** programmed to find the exact address of a tumor. Instead of dropping off packages at every house in the city (like chemotherapy does throughout the body), these drones fly straight to the cancer site and unload their cargo —whether it's medicine, gene silencers, or cancer-killing viruses.

Why This Is Encouraging for Patients

1. **Targeted Attack, Fewer Side Effects**
   MSCs can navigate directly to tumors, acting like precision-guided missiles, reducing damage to the rest of the body.
2. **Empowering the Immune System**
   Instead of treating cancer only with toxic chemicals, these engineered MSCs can deliver signals that rally the body's defenses—making treatment more natural and sustainable.
3. **Deep-Tissue Reach**
   Stem cells can penetrate hard-to-reach or metastatic tumors, potentially treating cancers that are historically difficult to manage.
4. **Building Toward Clinical Use**
   These studies are not just scientific curiosities—they represent real progress toward treatments that could soon be applied in humans, with an increased focus on both **efficacy** and **safety**.

Each of these advances brings us closer to a future where MSCs serve as smart, self-guided therapies—seeking out cancer, delivering potent treatments, and empowering the patient's biology to help in recovery. The ongoing work, especially in 2024–2025, showcases a field alive with promise and movement toward real-world impact.

6.3 Awakening the Immune System with Stem Cells

Cancer is skilled at hiding from our immune system. It cloaks itself to avoid detection—like a wolf in sheep's clothing. The exciting promise of stem cell therapy lies in its ability to **detect cancer and reawaken our body's natural defenses.**

How Stem Cells Can Help the Immune System Fight Cancer

1. **Targeted Cytokine Delivery**
   Stem cells, particularly MSCs, can be engineered to release **cytokines**—special proteins that alert and activate immune cells—directly in the tumor environment. This localized signal can help immune cells recognize and eliminate cancer cells with much lower risk of side effects than systemic therapies. A 2024 springboard review highlights MSCs' ability to regulate the immune system, target tumors, and deliver therapeutic molecules safely [114].
2. **Combining Resources with Immunotherapy**
   When paired with existing immunotherapies, such as checkpoint inhibitors (e.g., anti-PD-1), MSCs can significantly enhance treatment outcomes. A 2025 study found that engineered MSCs may enhance immune responses and tumor targeting when used in conjunction with immunotherapy drugs—a powerful synergy to overcome cancer's defenses [115].
3. **Overcoming Immune Resistance**
   Cancer stem cells (CSCs) can hide from immune attack by adapting to evade detection. New reviews emphasize the need to target these CSCs in immunotherapy models to prevent therapy resistance and relapse [116].

Why This Matters

- **Precision immune activation:** Instead of flooding the body with cytokines, stem cells deliver the signal exactly where needed—at the tumor—minimizing systemic harm.

- **Turning the tide in early trials:** Many current immunotherapy breakthroughs now incorporate stem cell strategies to prime the immune system more effectively.
- **A hopeful pathway forward:** The combination of stem cells with immune therapies is creating more adaptable, effective, and less toxic cancer treatments.

Summary Table

Benefit	What It Means for Patients
Targeted action	Fewer side effects, less damage to healthy tissue
Synergistic therapies	Enhances power of existing immunotherapy treatments
Long-lasting immune memory	Potentially reduces relapse and enhances quality of life

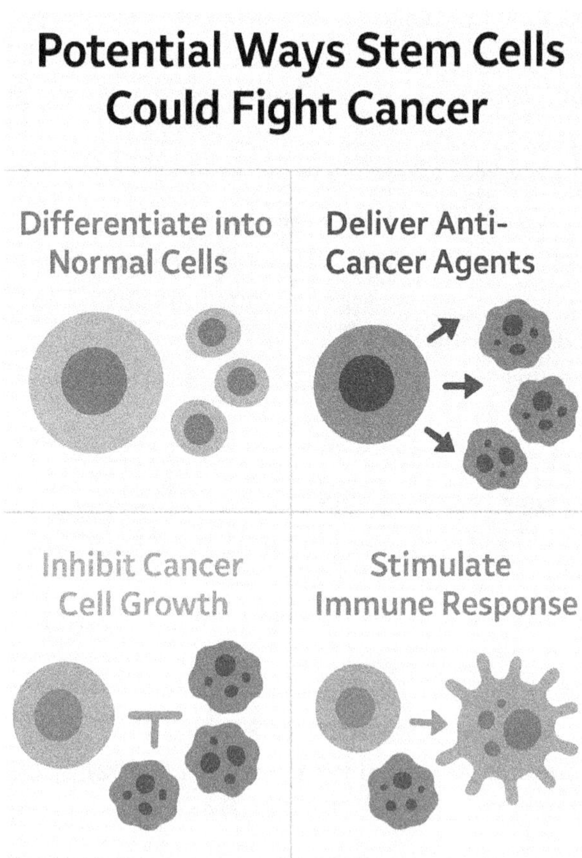

6.4 Healing the Body: How Stem Cells Help Repair Treatment Damage

While traditional treatments save lives, they often leave behind scars on the body. Cancer treatments like chemotherapy and radiotherapy are powerful —but they don't just target cancer cells; they can also harm healthy tissues. Radiation, for example, can damage skin, intestines, or salivary glands, while chemotherapy can weaken the heart or lungs. Days, weeks, or months after treatment, patients may experience lingering damage to organs such as the gastrointestinal tract, salivary glands, or skin, which can impact their quality of life.

Researchers are now testing whether stem cells can be used as the body's own **repair crew**, helping to rebuild these damaged tissues. Early studies suggest that MSCs may be able to reduce inflammation, encourage healing, and restore function in organs injured during cancer therapy, offering patients not only survival but also a better quality of life.

Key Ways Stem Cells Aid Recovery

1. Healing the Gut After Chemotherapy

Chemotherapy can damage the intestinal lining, leading to pain, nutrient malabsorption, and an increased risk of infection. A recent study found that MSCs can encourage the regrowth of the intestinal epithelium (the lining), helping restore function and comfort quickly [117].

2. Restoring Salivary Gland Function After Radiation

Head and neck cancer patients often suffer from chronic dry mouth (xerostomia) due to radiation damage. A 2025 follow-up study showed that injecting adipose-derived MSCs into salivary glands significantly reduced dry-mouth symptoms and improved quality of life—though more research is needed to confirm long-term effects [118].

3. Easing Radiation-Induced Lung Injury

Lungs exposed to radiation—especially during treatment for chest cancers —can develop complications like pneumonitis or fibrosis. While clinical trials are still pending, a growing body of laboratory evidence suggests that MSCs may reduce inflammation and promote lung tissue regeneration [119, 120].

4. Healing Radiation Skin Injuries

In a promising new initiative, the International Atomic Energy Agency (IAEA) is funding research into MSC-based therapies to repair severe radiation-induced skin damage—offering hope to patients recovering from accidental or therapeutic irradiation [121].

Why Patients and Families Can Feel Hopeful

- **Targeted Healing:** Unlike broad supportive treatments, stem cells seek out injury sites to promote healing directly where the damage is, helping tissues recover faster.
- **Symptom Relief:** Improvements in chronic symptoms—such as dry mouth or gut discomfort—can support better hydration, eating habits, and overall well-being.
- **Improved Quality of Life:** Patients report restored energy, reduced pain, and a greater return to normal activities.
- **Innovation in Progress:** These therapies are rapidly moving from lab research to clinical testing—bringing real, regenerative hope sooner.

6.5 Targeting Cancer Stem Cells: Striking at the Root of the Problem

Cancer stem cells (CSCs) are a rare yet highly aggressive type of cancer cell. Think of them as the **master seeds** of a tumor—able to grow into many kinds of cancer cells, survive treatments that kill most of the tumor, and start the disease again later. This is why some cancers come back months or even years after apparently successful therapy.

Unlike most cancer cells, CSCs can **self-renew** (make copies of themselves indefinitely) and **differentiate** (create various cell types within the tumor). They're also experts at hiding from the immune system and resisting chemotherapy and radiotherapy. Because of this, many researchers believe that truly curing cancer means finding ways to **eliminate CSCs.**

How Stem Cells Could Help Defeat CSCs

Scientists are exploring several MSC-based strategies to hunt down and neutralize CSCs:

1. **Delivering Precision Drugs to CSCs**
   MSCs can be engineered to carry drugs or small molecules that specifically bind to **CSC markers**—proteins found on their surface, such

as CD44, CD133, and ALDH1. This means the treatment can detect CSCs even when they are hidden deep within the tumor [106, 122].

2. **Shutting Down CSC Survival Signals**
   CSCs rely on specific **molecular signaling pathways**—like Wnt/β-catenin, Notch, and Hedgehog—to stay alive and maintain their stem-like properties. MSCs can be used to deliver inhibitors that block these pathways, making CSCs more vulnerable to destruction [123, 124].
3. **Boosting Immune Recognition of CSCs**
   One reason CSCs are hard to kill is that the immune system often ignores them. MSCs can be programmed to secrete cytokines such as IL-15 or GM-CSF that "flag" CSCs for attack by immune cells. Combining MSC therapy with cancer vaccines may also help the body remember and target CSCs in the future [125, 126].

Why This Matters for Long-Term Remission

Most conventional therapies focus on reducing tumor size quickly—but if CSCs survive, they can quietly regrow the tumor. By targeting CSCs directly, researchers aim for **deep, lasting remissions** and possibly complete cures. This is particularly important in aggressive cancers like glioblastoma, pancreatic cancer, and triple-negative breast cancer, where relapse rates remain high.

6.6 Preventing Recurrence and Metastasis

One of the biggest fears for cancer survivors is that the disease might return (recurrence) or spread to new parts of the body (metastasis). Even when scans show no visible tumors, tiny clusters of cancer cells—sometimes called *minimal residual disease*—can hide in tissues for months or years. These cells can later "wake up" and cause the cancer to come back. Preventing this from happening is one of the most critical frontiers in cancer research.

How MSC-Based Therapies May Help

Scientists are exploring the use of mesenchymal stem cell (MSC)-based therapies as a form of "maintenance therapy"—a long-term strategy aimed at keeping cancer away after initial treatment.

1. Periodic MSC Infusions

- Engineered MSCs could be given at intervals (for example, every few months) after standard cancer treatment.
- These MSCs might be modified to:
    1. Seek out hidden cancer cells anywhere in the body.
    2. Release targeted anti-cancer drugs, immune-activating molecules, or genetic "instructions" that push cancer cells into self-destruction.
- Early laboratory studies suggest that this approach could reduce the risk of relapse by **continuously monitoring the body** for occult cancer cells [101, 127].

2. MSC-Based Imaging Agents

- MSCs can be labeled with safe, traceable markers that show up in highly sensitive scans (such as PET or MRI).
- Because MSCs naturally travel to areas of disease, this method could detect cancer spread **before it becomes visible** on conventional scans—sometimes months earlier.

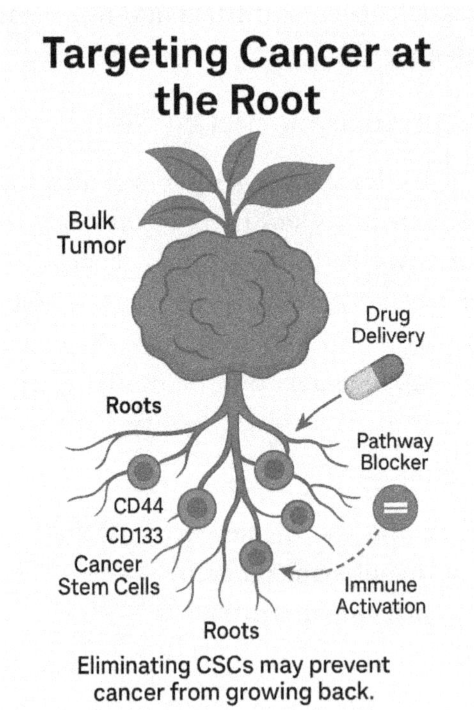

Stem Cells Could be Combined With Other New Technologies

Stem cell research doesn't stand alone—it is increasingly being combined with other cutting-edge technologies. For example, scientists are testing stem cells in conjunction with **immunotherapy**, which enhances the immune system's ability to fight cancer, or using **gene editing tools** like CRISPR to make stem cells more powerful and precise. Others are pairing stem cells with **nanotechnology**, creating ultra-tiny carriers that can be loaded into stem cells for even sharper tumor targeting. These combinations hold the promise of therapies that are not just powerful but **personalized** for each patient.

Emerging studies are demonstrating how MSCs can be engineered as 'Trojan horses'—carrying imaging markers or therapeutic payloads straight to tumor sites, enabling both detection and treatment simultaneously" [128]. In glioblastoma models, MSCs carrying imaging genes have been used successfully for non-invasive tumor tracking and therapy guidance [129]. Moreover, new insights into MSC kinetics and behavior are essential for designing safe and effective delivery approaches. This could allow doctors to intervene much sooner, when the cancer is still microscopic and far easier to treat.

Key Facts
Some studies combine stem cells with nanotechnology for precision therapy.

Why This Approach is Promising

- **Precision targeting** – MSCs home directly to tumor sites, meaning treatment is focused on dangerous cells and less likely to harm healthy tissues.
- **Reduced toxicity** – Unlike prolonged chemotherapy, MSC maintenance therapy could have fewer side effects, making it more tolerable for long-term use.
- **Proactive care** – Instead of waiting for cancer to return, doctors could stay one step ahead.

> ***A Patient's Perspective:*** *I*magine Luise, a breast cancer survivor whose greatest fear is that her cancer might come back. She joins a trial for MSC maintenance therapy. Every three months, she receives a quick infusion. The cells are engineered to hunt for any cancer hiding in her body. *"It feels like having a security system inside me,"* Luise says. *"It's given me peace of mind that I never thought I'd have again."*

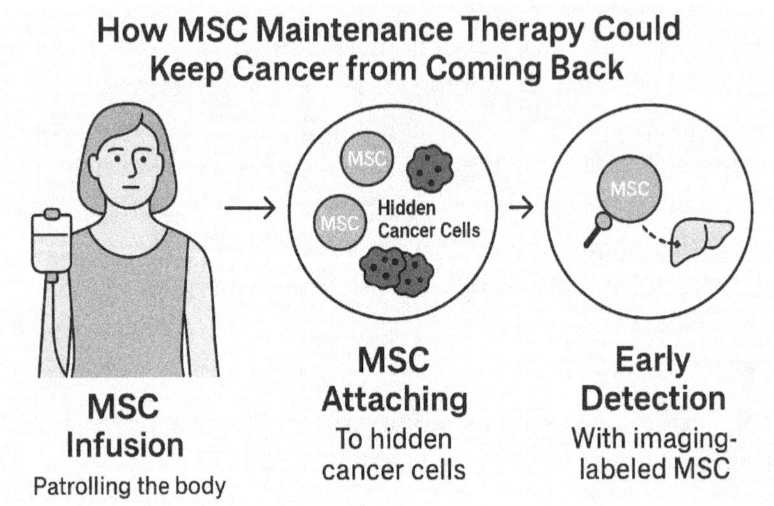

Challenges Ahead

- Researchers still need to prove that MSC maintenance therapy truly prevents recurrence in humans.
- The best cell dose, infusion schedule, and engineering strategy are still being studied.
- Clinical trials are ongoing, and results from large-scale studies are expected in the coming years.

6.7 Current Clinical Trials and Their Promise

As of 2024, **over 200 clinical trials worldwide are** exploring stem cell–based therapies in cancer care, ranging from delivering targeted treatments to aiding recovery after aggressive therapies [130]. Early findings are giving patients and researchers renewed hope.

What These Trials Are Reporting

- **Encouraging Safety Profiles**
  Multiple studies consistently affirm that **MSC therapies are safe**, with no serious side effects observed in most patients [131].
- **Faster Functional Recovery & Fewer Complications**
  Early-stage trials—like the REMODEL and REMEDY studies—highlight how MSC treatments can accelerate healing, particularly in conditions beyond cancer, laying the groundwork for oncology applications [132, 133].

- **Tumor Shrinkage and Extended Remissions (Preclinical and Early-Stage)**
  While large-scale cancer trials are still underway, initial findings suggest that MSCs—especially when engineered to deliver therapeutic agents—can help reduce tumor size and delay progression [101].

Looking Ahead: What Makes Us Hopeful

- **Broadening Clinical Testing**
  With hundreds of studies in progress, the patient populations, tumor types, and treatment strategies being tested are increasingly diverse.
- **Innovative Combination Therapies**
  Many trials now pair MSCs with advanced gene editing, biomaterial scaffolds, and AI-guided personalization—pushing the frontier of precision medicine [133].
- **Early Success Inspires Momentum**
  Even trials in unrelated fields (like GVHD or autoimmune diseases) demonstrate MSCs' effectiveness in modulating immune response and reducing inflammation—skills critical in cancer recovery as well.

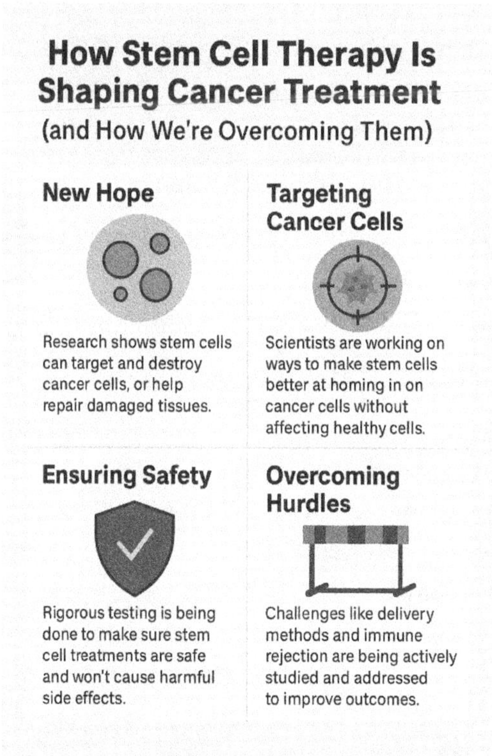

How Stem Cell Therapy Is Shaping Cancer Treatment
(and How We're Overcoming Them)
New Hope
Research shows stem cells can target and destroy cancer cells, or help repair damaged tissues.
Targeting Cancer Cells
Scientists are working on ways to make stem cells better at homing in on cancer cells without affecting healthy cells.
Ensuring Safety
Rigorous testing is being done to make sure stem cell treatments are safe and won't cause harmful side effects.
Overcoming Hurdles
Challenges like delivery methods and immune rejection are being actively studied and addressed to improve outcomes.

Snapshot Table: Early Cancer Trials with MSCs

Trial Focus	Early Outcomes	Next Steps
Safety evaluations	MSC therapies show high safety	Larger, Phase II/III trials upcoming
Supportive care post-treatment	Reports of faster healing, fewer side effects	Scaling to diverse patient groups
Direct tumor targeting	Tumor shrinkage in early studies	Better-engineered MSCs are under development
Regulatory validation	FDA approval in non-cancer use	Opens door for cancer-related approvals

Why This Matters for Patients and Families

1. **More Treatment Options**
   Patients facing aggressive or recurrent cancers may soon have access to new therapies that are both effective and better tolerated.
2. **Improved Life Quality**
   MSCs offer the promise of fewer toxic effects and faster functional recovery—giving back energy, comfort, and hope.
3. **Foundations for the Future**
   Each success, each trial advances the global understanding of stem cell therapy—paving the way for safer, more innovative cancer treatments ahead.

6.8 Challenges and Safety Considerations

Stem cell therapies—especially those involving MSCs—hold immense promise in the fight against cancer. Yet, as with any powerful tool, they come with challenges that researchers are working to address carefully.

1. Could MSCs Unintentionally Support Cancer?

While MSCs can fight cancer, under certain conditions, they might encourage tumors to grow. Recent findings show that:

- MSCs can suppress the activity of T cells and natural killer (NK) cells, weakening the immune system's ability to attack cancer and potentially allowing tumors to thrive.
- MSCs may also transform into **carcinoma-associated fibroblasts (CAFs)** within the tumor's surrounding environment. These CAFs can support the

tumor's growth and help new blood vessels form (angiogenesis), providing the tumor with nutrients and oxygen [115, 130]

This dual nature—potentially both cancer-fighting and cancer-promoting—underscores the importance of precisely engineering and regulating the behavior of MSCs.

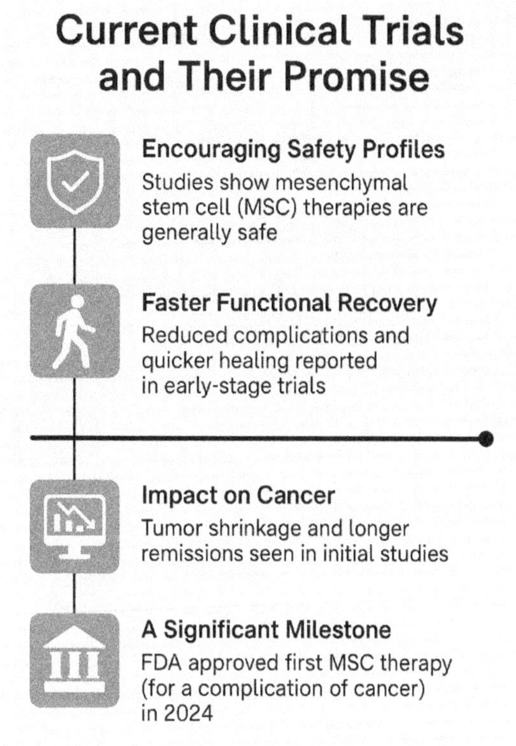

2. Immune Reactions and Graft Rejection

Although MSCs generally avoid strong immune reactions, there's still a risk of rejection—especially with **allogeneic MSCs** (stem cells from donors). The body's immune surveillance may recognize and clear them, and preexisting antibodies can block their function.

3. Variability in Potency and Poor Engraftment

Not all MSC batches perform equally:

- Cells sourced from different donors or tissue types (such as bone marrow versus fat) can vary significantly in potency.
- In some clinical trials, MSCs have failed to integrate effectively into target tissues, reducing their therapeutic impact [134].

To overcome this, researchers are exploring the use of CRISPR-engineered MSCs and biomaterial scaffolds to enhance cell viability and consistency.

4. Manufacturing Complexity and Cost

Producing MSC therapies is a complex and expensive process. It involves:

- Harvesting cells (sometimes via invasive procedures like bone marrow extraction)
- Cultivating them under strict lab conditions (GMP standards)
- Rigorous quality checks, purification, and storage protocols

The entire process requires sophisticated infrastructure and remains costly —especially for personalized (autologous) treatments [135, 136].

5. Supply Chain and Logistical Challenges

The process of delivering viable stem cells safely to patients involves:

- Coordinating cold storage, blood banks, and transport systems
- Ensuring a consistent supply amid external disruptions like pandemics or regulatory changes
- Managing logistics across countries and healthcare systems

Balancing Risks and Rewards

Despite these challenges, ongoing research is actively addressing them:

- Genetic and bioengineering strategies are being tested to ensure MSCs target tumors precisely without supporting them.
- Regulatory frameworks for cell therapy manufacturing are evolving to improve consistency and reduce costs.
- Advances in automation, AI-driven cell selection, and manufacturing technology are paving the way for safer, scalable, and more affordable treatments.

Challenge	Why It Matters	Potential Solutions
Tumor promotion risk	Could worsen cancer if MSCs act like CAFs	Better MSC engineering and control of differentiation
Immune rejection	Therapy fails if MSCs are cleared	Improved cell matching and immune cloaking
Inconsistent potency	Variable and unreliable results	Standardization and cell quality assessment
High cost and complexity	Limits patient access	Automation and process streamlining
Logistical hurdles	Delays impact therapy availability	Optimized supply chain and regulatory support

Why This Matters

Understanding these challenges doesn't dampen the promise of MSC therapies—it sharpens it. As technologies advance, the aim is to deliver powerful but safe treatments that are accessible to all who need them. With each hurdle surmounted, MSC-based therapies move closer to becoming practical, life-saving medicine in the lab.

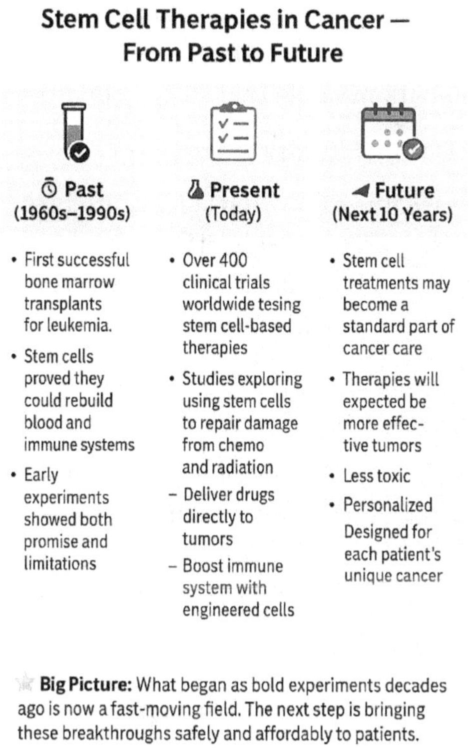

6.9 Looking Ahead: A More Hopeful Future

The field of stem cell research in cancer treatment is advancing at a breathtaking pace, and for patients, this means one thing: **hope is growing stronger every day**. What once seemed like a distant dream—personalized, gentle, and highly effective cancer treatments—is now beginning to take shape in laboratories and early clinical trials worldwide.

Precision Medicine Becomes Personal

Imagine a future where your cancer treatment is designed just for you—tailored not only to your cancer type but to your genetic blueprint. With stem cell–based therapies, doctors could use your cells, reprogrammed and enhanced, to fight cancer with pinpoint accuracy. This approach could minimize harmful side effects while maximizing the cancer-killing effect.

Powerful Combination Therapies

Rather than replacing existing treatments, stem cell therapy could work hand-in-hand with immunotherapy, targeted drugs, and radiation. Like members of an elite rescue team, each treatment would play its role—stem cells homing in on tumors, immune therapies activating your body's defenses, and targeted drugs attacking cancer at the molecular level. Together, these combinations could dramatically improve survival rates.

Making Cancer Care More Comfortable

Right now, cancer treatments often mean frequent hospital visits, prolonged infusions, and complex side effects. However, it's possible that specially engineered stem cells could be administered in outpatient clinics—or perhaps even at home—making cancer care more convenient and less disruptive to daily life.

Why There's a Real Reason for Optimism

In the past five years, the number of clinical trials involving stem cells for cancer has more than doubled. Early results are showing not only safety but also encouraging signs of effectiveness—patients recovering faster after chemotherapy, tumors shrinking in hard-to-treat cancers, and immune systems bouncing back stronger than before [107]

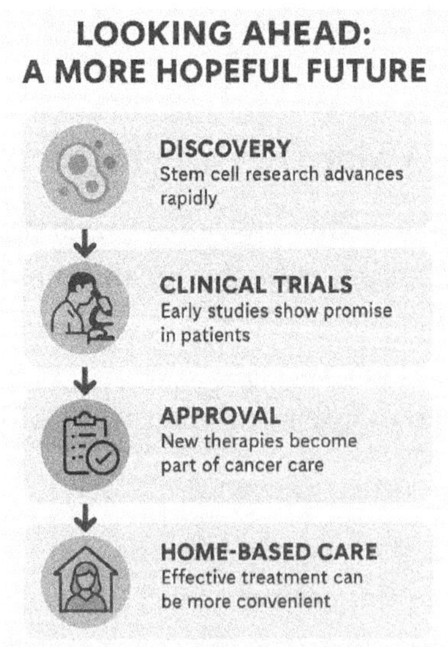

Chapter 7 – Stem Cells in Clinical Trials

When people hear the words *"clinical trial,"* it can sound intimidating or overly scientific. However, in reality, clinical trials are the method by which doctors and researchers carefully test new treatments to determine if they are safe, effective, and beneficial for patients. Without them, no new medicine or therapy could ever reach the hospital or clinic. Stem cell research is no exception—before any stem cell-based cancer therapy can be widely used, it must go through this rigorous process.

Clinical trials represent the bridge between promising ideas in the lab and real therapies for people with cancer. They are where hope and science meet.

> ***Patient Quote:*** *"At first, I worried about being a 'test subject.' However, I then realized that clinical trials are the primary method by which new treatments are discovered. By joining one, I was helping myself—and helping science."* — Maria, 42.

7.1 What Are Clinical Trials?

A clinical trial is like a carefully designed experiment involving people, rather than test tubes or lab animals. They are guided by strict ethical rules and monitored by independent committees to ensure patient protection.

The process is divided into **phases**, each with a specific goal:

- **Phase I:** Tests safety. A small group of patients receives the treatment to determine if it is tolerated and to assess for potential side effects.
- **Phase II:** Tests effectiveness. Researchers investigate whether the treatment is effective against cancer in a larger patient population.

- **Phase III**: Compares the new treatment to the current "standard of care" in hundreds or thousands of patients. If successful, the therapy may be approved for medical use.
- **Phase IV**: This phase occurs after approval, involving monitoring how the treatment works in everyday clinics and hospitals.

Think of these phases as checkpoints. Only when a therapy passes one phase can it move forward. This way, by the time it reaches the wider public, patients and doctors can be confident that it has undergone thorough testing.

> ***Did You Know?***
> The first successful **bone marrow transplant** was performed in 1956 between identical twins. Today, over 1 million stem cell transplants have been performed worldwide.

> ***A Patient's Story:*** Maria, a 42-year-old teacher, was diagnosed with lymphoma. Standard chemotherapy worked at first, but her cancer returned. When her doctors suggested a **stem cell clinical trial**, she hesitated—after all, who wants to feel like a "guinea pig"?
>
> But she soon learned an important truth: trials aren't experiments on people; they are experiments for people. Every safeguard was in place: strict monitoring, clear consent forms, and a dedicated medical team.
>
> Maria enrolled in a Phase II study using **hematopoietic stem cells (HSCs)** from cord blood. After undergoing high-dose chemotherapy to clear her bone marrow, she received the transplant. Recovery wasn't instant—it was slow and sometimes frustrating. But six months later, her scans showed no evidence of cancer.

Maria isn't just grateful for her second chance; she's proud to be part of research that may help countless other patients in the future. Her story is one of many showing how clinical trials are not only about science, but also about human courage and hope.

> ***Did You Know?***
> Every patient in a clinical trial contributes to medical progress—even if the treatment doesn't work for them. Data from "unsuccessful" trials often guide the next breakthrough.

7.2 Examples of Stem Cell Trials in Cancer

Stem cells are being investigated in various ways to aid cancer patients. Here are some examples that illustrate both progress and promise:

- **Hematopoietic stem cell transplants** are already standard for blood cancers like leukemia, lymphoma, and multiple myeloma. Decades of clinical trials transformed bone marrow and cord blood transplants into lifesaving procedures, restoring healthy blood and immune cells after chemotherapy or radiation.
- **Mesenchymal stem cells.** Some trials are exploring how MSCs might deliver anti-cancer drugs directly to tumors, acting like "biological couriers." Others are testing their ability to reduce the harmful side effects of chemotherapy, such as inflammation or organ damage.
- **Experimental gene-edited stem cells.** In a few cutting-edge trials, researchers are using tools like CRISPR to improve stem cells—making them more resistant to cancer or better at supporting the immune system [137].
- **Combination approaches.** Some trials are pairing stem cells with **immunotherapy** (treatments that boost the immune system) to attack cancer more effectively.

Did You Know?

More than 6,000 clinical trials worldwide currently include the word "stem cells" in their registration. These trials explore many possibilities—from repairing heart damage to treating neurological diseases.. Still, the number of cancer-related stem cell studies is rising every year. This rapid growth demonstrates the high hopes scientists have for stem cells and the fast pace at which the field is advancing toward real medical breakthroughs.

7.3 Successes and Setbacks

Like all areas of medicine, progress comes with both victories and lessons learned:

- **Successes:** HSC transplants are among the clearest examples of stem cells saving lives. Tens of thousands of patients worldwide have benefited. Clinical studies also demonstrate that stem cells can help mitigate complications following cancer therapy, thereby accelerating recovery and enhancing quality of life [138].
- **Setbacks:** Not every trial succeeds. Some MSC studies have shown mixed results—sometimes the cells helped, other times they seemed to protect tumors instead of fighting them. These mixed outcomes remind scientists to proceed with caution and underscore the importance of strict clinical testing.

Every result—whether positive or negative—teaches researchers something valuable and helps shape safer, better treatments for the future.

> *Did You Know?*
> Only about **1 in 10 experimental cancer therapies** that enter Phase I trials eventually reach approval. That's why patience, persistence, and many parallel trials are needed.

7.4 Why This Matters for Patients

For patients, clinical trials mean two things: **hope** and **caution**.

- **Hope:** New therapies are being tested every year, and many offer real promise for patients whose cancers are hard to treat.
- **Caution:** Not every clinic advertising "stem cell cures" is part of a legitimate trial. Proper clinical trials are carefully registered, monitored, and often provided at no cost to participants.

If you or someone you know is interested in exploring stem cell therapies, a trusted resource is: euclinicaltrials.eu or ClinicalTrials.gov, where you can find official listings of ongoing studies. Many cancer centers also have patient navigators who can explain trial options.

> *Did You Know?*
> Legitimate clinical trials are usually **free to patients**—in fact, many cover travel and treatment costs. If a clinic requests large payments, it's a warning sign.

7.5 An Optimistic Outlook

Although challenges remain, each trial brings us one step closer to safer and more powerful stem cell–based cancer treatments. The journey from the lab to the clinic may be long, but history has already shown us that stem cell therapies can move from experimental ideas to treatments.

Stories like Maria's remind us: behind every statistic and trial number, **there is a real person** whose life may be transformed—not just by science, but by hope.

Patient Tip Box: Considering a Stem Cell Clinical Trial?

If you or a loved one is thinking about joining a clinical trial, here are some helpful questions and reminders:

Questions to Ask Your Doctor

- What is the **goal** of this trial—safety, effectiveness, or comparison to standard treatment?

- What **phase** is the trial in?
- What are the possible **benefits and risks** for me personally?
- Will I still receive standard treatment, or will I only accept the experimental therapy?
- How will my health be monitored during the trial?
- Are there **costs** involved, or is the trial covered by the sponsor?

Red Flags to Watch Out For

- Clinics are requesting **large upfront payments** (legitimate trials are typically free).
- Promises of a guaranteed "**cure.**"
- No listing on trusted registries, such as euclinicaltrials.eu or ClinicalTrials.gov.
- There is no clear explanation of **ethics committee oversight**.

Remember

Clinical trials are designed to protect patients while exploring new frontiers of medicine. Asking the right questions helps ensure you're participating in safe, well-regulated research that could benefit both you and future patients.

Part III: Real-World Impact and Future Directions

Chapter 8 – What Patients Should Know

When faced with a cancer diagnosis, it's natural to want to explore every possible treatment option. The news can feel overwhelming, and patients often describe it as being suddenly thrown into a storm—one where every decision feels urgent and every choice feels like it could change the outcome. In this search for hope, it's only natural to look beyond standard treatments and wonder about new possibilities, especially those often featured in the headlines.

Stem cell therapies are among the most talked-about advances in modern medicine. They frequently appear in news stories, on websites, and even in advertisements that promise cures for diseases once thought to be untreatable. Many patients and families wonder: *Could stem cells help me? Could this be the breakthrough I've been waiting for?*

The truth is both exciting and complicated. Stem cell research holds enormous promise, but it is also an area where **hope and hype can sometimes become intertwined.** On the one hand, decades of rigorous scientific research have already led to proven, lifesaving stem cell treatments, especially for blood cancers. On the other hand, some clinics and companies exploit patients' fears and hopes, offering unproven therapies that lack evidence-based support.

> ***Patient Quote***: *"When I was first diagnosed, the first thing I did was Google stem cells. I found pages full of promises and success stories. It gave me hope, but also confusion—how could I tell what was real and what wasn't?"* — Anna, 50.

Anna's words reflect what so many patients feel: curiosity, hope, and sometimes vulnerability in the face of too much information.

That's why it is so crucial for patients and families to understand what stem cell science can and cannot yet deliver. This chapter is here to help you **separate fact from fiction**, to explain the real benefits and risks clearly, and to give you the tools to ask the right questions. With the proper knowledge, you can make informed choices—not just out of fear or urgency, but with confidence, caution, and realistic hope.

8.1 Hope vs. Hype

When people hear about stem cells in the news, it's often presented as something almost magical—cells that can turn into many different tissues, heal the body, and maybe even cure diseases once thought untreatable. It's easy to see why patients with cancer and their families feel hopeful. And indeed, there is real reason for hope.

Stem cell therapies are already part of everyday medicine. For example, **hematopoietic stem cell (HSC) transplants**, also known as bone marrow or blood stem cell transplants, are routinely used for patients with leukemia, lymphoma, and multiple myeloma [138]. These treatments can completely rebuild a patient's blood and immune system after intensive chemotherapy or radiation. For many people, they have been life-saving. That's not hype—that's proven medical progress.

But alongside genuine breakthroughs, there's also a lot of noise. Some private clinics advertise stem cell treatments as if they were miracle cures for nearly everything—from cancer to Alzheimer's disease to aging itself. These treatments often come with a high price tag and minimal scientific backing. Websites may feature glowing testimonials, but if there's no peer-reviewed evidence, no clinical trial registration, and no oversight by medical authorities, patients are essentially being asked to take a gamble with their health.

The danger of hype is that it **preys on hope**. When someone is vulnerable, especially during a *cancer journey*, the promise of an easy cure can be incredibly tempting. But while experimental therapies are worth exploring through safe, regulated trials, jumping into unproven clinics can lead to disappointment, wasted money, or even harm.

The reality is more nuanced than either of these extremes. Stem cells are not magic bullets—but neither are they science fiction. They are powerful biological tools that scientists are learning to use more wisely every year.

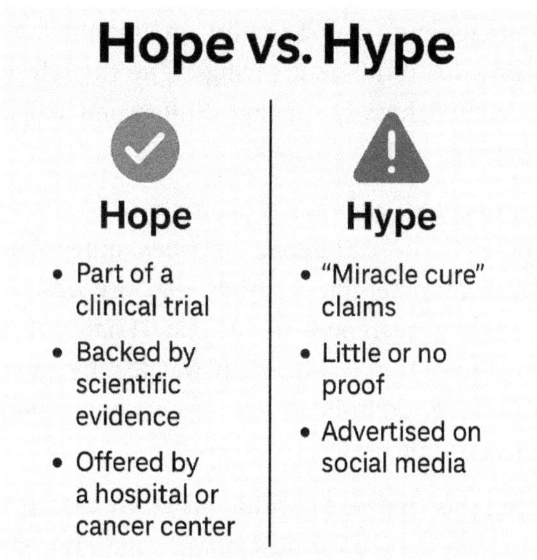
Hope vs. Hype
Hope
• Part of a clinical trial
• Backed by scientific evidence
• Offered by a hospital or cancer center
Hype
• "Miracle cure" claims
• Little or no proof
• Advertised on social media

The truth lies between **unrealistic promises** and **discouraging skepticism**: progress is real, but it takes time, careful testing, and honesty about both successes and setbacks.

For patients and their families, the key is to celebrate genuine hope while recognizing the signs of hype. If something sounds too good to be true, it probably is. But if it's part of a clinical trial, backed by scientific publications, and offered at a respected hospital or cancer center, then it's worth genuine attention.

In short
Hope is real, but it grows incrementally. By learning to distinguish between reliable science and empty promises, patients can protect themselves while remaining open to breakthroughs that truly change lives.

8.2 A Patient's Story: James's Choice

James, a 58-year-old father of three, had already endured months of chemotherapy for his lymphoma. The treatments had left him exhausted, with thinning hair and low energy, but he was determined to fight for more time with his family. While searching online late at night, James came across a private clinic advertising a **"stem cell cure for cancer."** The website was filled with glowing testimonials and hopeful promises. Smiling patients claimed they had been "cured," yet when James looked closer, he found **no published studies, no clinical trial registration, and no mention of oversight by medical authorities.**

The price tag was staggering—over **$40,000**, an amount James would have had to borrow against his retirement savings. The thought of draining his family's finances weighed heavily on him. Still, when you are desperate, even slim promises can seem like lifelines.

Fortunately, James decided to bring the brochure to his oncologist. His doctor gently explained the difference between unregulated treatments sold for profit and legitimate clinical trials that are designed to protect patients. Together, they searched the ClinicalTrials.gov database and discovered a nearby Phase II trial. The study was testing mesenchymal stem cells (MSCs) to reduce complications after chemotherapy, such as inflammation and tissue damage.

Unlike the fake clinic, this trial was **conducted at no cost**. It was funded by research grants, approved by an ethics board, and staffed by a team of doctors, nurses, and researchers who carefully monitored every participant. James felt reassured knowing he would be in safe hands, with his health tracked at every step.

By joining the trial, James did more than seek care for himself—he became part of a scientific effort that could help countless future patients. He avoided the risk of an unproven, expensive treatment and instead contributed to research that may one day make cancer therapy safer and more effective.

James's story is a reminder that **hope is real, but it must be guided by evidence.** Asking questions, checking sources, and trusting therapies backed by solid science can mean the difference between taking a dangerous gamble and opening the door to genuine progress.

Questions James Asked His Doctor

When James was unsure whether to trust a private clinic or consider a clinical trial, these were the key questions he brought to his oncologist:

✓ **Is this treatment part of a registered clinical trial?**
 – If not, why not?

✓ **What scientific evidence supports it?**
 – Are there peer-reviewed studies in medical journals?

✓ **Who is overseeing the trial or treatment?**
 – Is there an ethics board or regulatory agency involved?

✓**What are the possible risks and benefits?**

– How will side effects be managed?

✓**What are the costs?**

– Is it free as part of a study, or does the clinic expect large payments?

✓**Are there alternatives?**

– What standard treatments or other trials are available for my cancer?

Tip

Bringing these questions to your doctor can help protect you from false promises and guide you toward safe, evidence-based options.

8.3 Understanding the Benefits and Risks

Like all medical treatments, stem cell therapies bring both **tangible benefits** and **real risks**. For patients with certain blood cancers, a **hematopoietic stem cell transplant** may offer the chance of long-term remission—or even a cure. These transplants have saved thousands of lives worldwide and remain one of the most successful examples of stem cells already being used in modern medicine.

But these procedures are not simple. Before receiving the new stem cells, patients usually undergo **high-dose chemotherapy or radiation**. This process clears out diseased bone marrow, allowing new stem cells to settle in and begin producing healthy blood cells. While necessary, this preparatory step can be taxing on the body and carries short-term side effects, including fatigue, nausea, hair loss, and increased vulnerability to infections.

Common Risks Patients Face

- **Infections:** Because the immune system is temporarily "wiped clean," even a small cold or minor cut can turn serious. Patients are carefully monitored and often placed in special protective environments during this period.
- **Graft-versus-host disease (GVHD):** In **allogeneic transplants** (when stem cells are obtained from a donor), the new immune cells may mistakenly perceive the patient's body as foreign and attack it. Symptoms can range from mild rashes to severe damage to the liver, lungs, or intestines.
- **Organ damage and long-term complications:** The intensity of chemotherapy or radiation can, in some cases, cause heart, lung, or fertility problems later in life. Patients are followed closely for months or even years after their transplant to manage these risks.

The Benefits That Make It Worthwhile

Despite these challenges, the benefits can be profound. For many patients, a transplant offers the only chance of long-term survival. Once the new stem cells "engraft" and start working, they create a **new blood and immune system**—one that can recognize and attack lingering cancer cells. For some, this is the closest thing we have to a cure.

Where Research Is Headed

Scientists are working to make these treatments **safer and gentler**:

- **Mesenchymal stem cells** are being investigated as a means to modulate immune system overreactions, potentially reducing the risk of GVHD [139].
- **Reduced-intensity conditioning:** Some centers are experimenting with lower doses of chemotherapy or radiation before transplants, making the procedure less toxic for older patients or those with fragile health.
- **Better donor matching and cord blood banks:** Improvements in genetic matching reduce the risk of complications and make transplants more accessible to a broader range of people.

Striking the Balance

For patients, it's important to remember both sides of the equation. Stem cell therapies offer **real hope**, but they also carry significant risks. Doctors weigh each patient's unique situation—age, overall health, type of cancer—before recommending a transplant.

The bottom line: stem cell treatments are neither miracle cures nor reckless experiments. They are powerful tools that are constantly being refined. The safest path forward is to embrace both **the promise of progress** and **the honesty about risks**, so that every decision is made with eyes wide open.

Did You Know?
Every year, doctors perform more than **50,000 stem cell transplants worldwide**—most of them for blood cancers such as leukemia, lymphoma, and multiple myeloma. What began as an experimental idea in the 1960s has now become a routine, life-saving treatment for thousands of patients each year.

8.4 Clinical Trials: The Right Path Forward

For patients curious about stem cell therapies beyond standard transplants, the **safest and most promising way forward is through a**

registered clinical trial. These studies are not just experiments—they are carefully designed steps that bring tomorrow's treatments closer to reality. Every significant advance in cancer care, from chemotherapy to immunotherapy, once passed through the clinical trial process. Stem cell research is now following that same pathway.

Clinical trials are built with **patients' safety at the center**. Before a trial begins, it must be reviewed and approved by independent ethics committees and health authorities. This ensures that patients are fully informed, that risks are minimized, and that every treatment is closely monitored. Far from being "guinea pigs," participants are **partners in discovery**, helping doctors and scientists learn what works best.

For patients, joining a trial can mean:

- **Early access** to innovative therapies that aren't yet widely available. And almost always with the guarantee of continuity of treatment, after approval by the regulatory authorities, at no economic cost to the patient.
- **Close medical supervision**, with frequent check-ins and thorough follow-up care.
- The knowledge that they are **contributing to future progress**, giving hope not only to themselves but also to others who may face the same diagnosis in years to come.

A Patient's Story: Ana's New Hope

Ana, a 45-year-old mother of two, had battled leukemia for years. After standard chemotherapy and a bone marrow transplant, her cancer returned. She felt exhausted—not only physically, but emotionally—wondering if she had run out of options.

Her doctor mentioned a new clinical trial testing **gene-edited hematopoietic stem cells**, designed to rebuild the immune system so it could better recognize and fight cancer cells. At first, Ana was hesitant. She feared being a "test subject." But after learning how closely patients in trials are monitored and reassured by the strict safety protocols, she decided to participate.

The process was not easy—there were frequent hospital visits and plenty of blood tests. But Ana also felt a sense of empowerment. She was not passively receiving treatment; she was actively contributing to the science that could help others like her. Six months later, her scans showed promising results, and while her journey continues, Ana says she feels something she hadn't felt in a long time: **hope grounded in science, not just wishful thinking.**

Exploring trial opportunities is easier than many think. Databases such as ClinicalTrials.gov list thousands of ongoing studies worldwide. Many cancer centers also have trial navigators or coordinators whose job is to match patients with studies suited to their condition. Talking with your oncologist is the best starting point—they can help determine whether a trial is a good fit for your medical needs and personal circumstances.

While not every patient will qualify for a trial, the very existence of so many studies is a sign of rapid progress. Each trial builds on the lessons of the last, moving us closer to safer, more effective therapies. What is experimental today could very well be tomorrow's standard treatment.

🌟 *For patients, this means hope is not abstract—it is happening right now in hospitals and research centers across the globe. By taking part in clinical trials, you are not only seeking care for yourself but also helping to shape the future of cancer treatment.*

Did You Know?
Most legitimate clinical trials are **free for patients** because governments, universities, or research organizations fund them. Many also help cover extra expenses, such as travel or lodging, so patients can participate without worrying about overwhelming costs.

Joining a trial doesn't just give you access to new therapies—it also means you're cared for by a team of doctors and nurses who provide **close monitoring and extra support** throughout the study. For many patients, this level of attention feels more reassuring than standard care.

🌟 *By joining a clinical trial, you're not only opening the door to a new treatment—you're also helping move science forward for future patients.*

8.5 How to Evaluate Stem Cell Clinics and Treatments

Due to the growing excitement around stem cells, many patients are encountering advertisements from private clinics that promise **"revolutionary cures."** These offers often appear on websites, social media platforms, or even in glossy brochures with smiling patients and bold claims. The language is usually very persuasive—words like *miracle, guaranteed, cutting-edge,* or *no side effects* are used to create hope and urgency. For patients and families already under stress, these promises can feel almost irresistible.

However, **not all clinics are legitimate**, and some can be risky. Unlike approved clinical trials, these private operations may not have gone through the careful safety checks that protect patients. Treatments may be offered without proper scientific backing, without oversight from ethics boards, and without long-term data to prove safety. In some cases, patients have spent large sums of money only to experience no benefit—or even harmful complications.

The good news is that you don't need to feel helpless when faced with these choices. Patients and families have more power than they may realize. By asking the right questions and knowing what to look for, you can **separate trustworthy opportunities from dangerous ones.**

Here are some key steps:

- **Look for clinical trial registration**: Safe and legitimate stem cell therapies are usually offered within the framework of an official trial (such as those listed on ClinicalTrails.gov or national registries). If a clinic cannot provide a registration number or approval details, it's a warning sign.
- **Ask about oversight**: Ethical stem cell research is constantly reviewed by independent experts—ethics committees, institutional review boards, or government agencies. These bodies exist to protect patients from unsafe or exploitative practices.
- **Check for published evidence**: A trustworthy clinic should be able to provide references to peer-reviewed scientific studies that support their approach. Personal testimonials or flashy websites are not enough.
- **Discuss risks honestly**: Every real medical treatment—especially in cancer—has potential side effects. If a clinic promises there are "no risks," this is misleading. Transparency is a hallmark of safety.
- **Evaluate costs**: Most genuine clinical trials do not charge patients for the treatment itself. Some even help cover travel or lodging expenses. If you are asked to pay tens of thousands of dollars upfront, the treatment is likely not legitimate.

Most importantly, remember that you are not alone. Doctors, patient advocacy groups, and cancer organizations can help guide you toward **safe and evidence-based options**. Choosing wisely is not about being fearful—

it's about being empowered. Every time a patient chooses a legitimate path, it strengthens the scientific community and brings us all closer to safe, reliable treatments.

The hopeful message is this: while unregulated clinics may try to take advantage of patients, there are more and more safe, legitimate opportunities emerging every year. By staying informed and asking the right questions, you can protect yourself and remain open to the fundamental breakthroughs that stem cell science is making possible.

A Patient's Story: Rosa's Turning Point

Rosa, a 62-year-old grandmother, had been living with multiple myeloma. After her initial treatments, she began searching online for "new cures." She came across a glossy advertisement from a private clinic claiming **"100% safe stem cell cancer cures with no side effects."** The price was high—over $30,000—but Rosa was tempted.

Before making arrangements, she showed the clinic's brochure to her daughter, who insisted they discuss it with her oncologist. The oncologist pointed out several red flags: no clinical trial registration, no peer-reviewed studies, and vague promises of miracle results. Instead, the oncologist suggested Rosa consider a Phase II clinical trial testing stem cells to reduce the side effects of chemotherapy.

Rosa chose the trial. Not only was it free of charge, but she also received **personalized monitoring** from a dedicated research team. The experience reassured her that she was in safe hands. While the trial was still experimental, Rosa felt hopeful knowing her participation could help shape safer treatments for future patients.

Her story highlights an important truth: **being cautious doesn't mean giving up hope—it means channeling hope in the safest, most effective direction.**

Recognizing Red Flags

- **High-pressure tactics**: "Sign up quickly before spaces run out!"
- **Cash-only treatments**: Legitimate hospitals use standard billing systems.
- **Miracle cure claims**: No therapy works 100% of the time, especially in cancer.

►**Lack of transparency**: If you can't find clear information, that's a warning.

An Empowering Perspective

While it may feel discouraging to learn that some clinics are misleading patients, the reality is that **you are not powerless**. By asking the right questions and insisting on evidence, you can protect yourself and your loved ones.

More importantly, by choosing **registered clinical trials and trusted medical centers**, you are supporting the kind of research that genuinely advances the field. Each safe choice patients make helps weaken the influence of questionable clinics and strengthens the pathway toward real, reliable therapies.

The hopeful message is this: you don't have to gamble to seek cutting-edge care. Legitimate options exist—and they continue to grow every year. Your best defense is knowledge, and your best ally is a medical team you can trust.

8.6 An Optimistic Outlook

It's easy to feel overwhelmed when reading about cancer treatments—especially when new therapies seem experimental or uncertain. But when we take a step back and look at the big picture, the progress in stem cell research is truly remarkable. Just a few decades ago, the idea of using stem cells to treat cancer was considered highly experimental. Today, **hematopoietic stem cell transplants** are routine, lifesaving therapies for blood cancers, and **hundreds of new trials** are underway to explore broader applications.

The pace of discovery is accelerating. Researchers are learning not only how to use stem cells to **rebuild the body after harsh treatments** like chemotherapy and radiation, but also how to **engineer them into active cancer fighters**—delivering drugs, boosting the immune system, or repairing organs damaged by therapy. What once sounded like science fiction is becoming reality in leading cancer centers around the world.

For patients, this means that **hope is no longer just in the distant future—it's already arriving step by step**. Each successful clinical trial adds a new layer of knowledge. Each patient who participates brings us closer to therapies that are **safer, less toxic, and more personal**. While no single breakthrough will solve everything overnight, the combined progress is building a future where cancer care looks very different from today.

Importantly, patients now play a more central role than ever. By joining clinical trials, asking the right questions, and advocating for safe, evidence-based care, they help shape the direction of research. Families, communities, and support groups amplify this impact by raising awareness and resources. Science alone doesn't move forward—**people do, together**.

👨‍⚕️ The most inspiring truth is this: what is experimental today can become tomorrow's standard treatment. Just as bone marrow transplants were once a daring experiment and are now routine, so too could stem cell–based therapies evolve into everyday options for millions. The road ahead is full of promise, and each step brings us closer to a time when stem cells are not only repairing damage but also helping us finally **turn the tide against cancer**.

Patient Takeaway · A Message of Hope

"Every breakthrough in cancer care began as an idea, tested step by step in people just like me, Stem cell research is moving quickly, and while it's not yet percfect, it offers real hope for the future. What feels experimental today may be the treatment that saves lives tomorrow. Hope isn't just a dream—it's progress in motion."

Remember: By staying informed, asking questions, and trusting science, you are not only caring for yourself—you are also helping to shape the future of cancer treatment for generations to come.

Chapter 9 – Ethical and Safety Questions

Stem cell therapies for cancer carry tremendous promise, but with new frontiers in medicine come new challenges. Patients and families often ask: *"Is it safe?" "Is it ethical?"* These are not just scientific questions—they are deeply human ones. They touch on trust, fairness, and the responsibility researchers and doctors have toward the people they serve.

This chapter explores the key **ethical and safety issues** surrounding stem cell use in cancer treatment, why they matter, and how the medical community is working to address them.

> ***Patient Quote:*** *"I remember thinking: if stem cells are so powerful, why aren't they offered everywhere already? My doctor explained it's about safety, and that gave me peace of mind."* — Omar, 63.

9.1 Why Safety Comes First

Every therapy—even well-established ones—carries risks. Stem cell treatments are no different. Some of the main safety concerns include:

- **Tumor formation**: Because stem cells can grow and multiply, scientists must be sure they do not form new tumors themselves. This is especially important with pluripotent stem cells (which can become many cell types).
- **Immune reactions**: In transplants, the immune system may attack donor cells (as in graft-versus-host disease), or donor cells may attack the patient's body.
- **Unknown long-term effects**: Stem cell therapies are still relatively new. Scientists need years of follow-up data to understand their lasting impact.

To address these concerns, every legitimate clinical trial includes **layers of safety monitoring**—from laboratory experiments to animal studies to small, carefully controlled early-phase trials before any treatment is tested on large groups of people.

✨ *The hopeful message is this: safety is not an afterthought—it is the foundation. Each new step in stem cell therapy is only taken once strict safety checks are passed.*

> 💡 *Did You Know?*
> Before any stem cell therapy reaches patients, it undergoes years of testing in the laboratory and in animals to ensure its safety. In fact, fewer than **1 in 10 potential treatments** make it from early testing to approval—but the ones that do are far safer because of this process.

✨ *Every checkpoint exists to protect patients while advancing progress.*

9.2 The Ethics of Stem Cell Use

Stem cell research has often been the subject of intense ethical debate, particularly when it involves **embryonic stem cells**. These cells are taken from very early-stage embryos. Because embryos represent potential human life, their use raises deep moral questions about when life begins and how it should be valued. For many people, this is a sensitive and personal issue, shaped by culture, religion, and individual beliefs.

The good news is that **in cancer therapy today, most research does not rely on embryonic stem cells**. Instead, scientists focus on two other types:

- **Adult stem cells** encompass hematopoietic stem cells (HSCs) derived from the bone marrow and mesenchymal stem cells (MSCs) obtained from tissues such as fat or the umbilical cord. These cells are already widely used in medicine, and their collection usually carries little ethical controversy.
- **Induced pluripotent stem cells (iPSCs)** are adult cells "reprogrammed" in the lab to act like embryonic stem cells. iPSCs can be created from a patient's own skin or blood cells, avoiding the need for embryos altogether. They offer the same scientific advantages as embryonic cells but without many of the moral dilemmas.

This shift toward adult stem cells and induced pluripotent stem cells (iPSCs) has significantly **reduced ethical conflicts** in cancer research. Patients and families can feel reassured that most of today's progress is being built on ethically acceptable foundations.

Still, stem cell therapies raise other critical ethical questions:

- **Informed Consent**: Every patient deserves to know exactly what they are agreeing to. This means understanding not just the potential benefits of a stem cell trial, but also its risks, uncertainties, and alternatives. Valid informed consent is not just paperwork—it is a conversation built on honesty and respect.
- **Equity of Access**: Stem cell therapies are often expensive and complex. Will they be available only to patients in wealthy countries or to those who can pay high prices? Or will they be developed in ways that make them accessible to people everywhere? Fair access is one of the most significant ethical challenges for the future.
- **Oversight of Clinics**: As we saw in Chapter 8, some private clinics exploit vulnerable patients by offering unproven, costly "stem cell cures." Ethically, this is unacceptable. Patients deserve protection through strict oversight, transparency, and enforcement of standards.

At the heart of all these issues is a simple principle: respect for human dignity. Ethical stem cell research means treating patients honestly, ensuring fairness in access, and building therapies on a foundation of safety and truth.

The hopeful perspective is this: **science is finding ways to move forward responsibly.** With adult stem cells and iPSCs leading the way, cancer research can progress rapidly while honoring ethical values that matter to patients and society alike.

Did You Know?

In 2012, the Nobel Prize in Medicine was awarded to scientists Shinya Yamanaka and John Gurdon for their discovery of how to create **induced pluripotent stem cells** (iPSCs)—adult cells that can be reprogrammed to behave like embryonic stem cells.

This breakthrough enabled researchers to study and utilize stem cells **without relying on embryos**, providing an ethical and widely accepted alternative. iPSCs are now at the heart of many cancer and regenerative medicine studies, providing science with powerful tools while alleviating moral concerns.

This demonstrates how innovation and ethics can advance in tandem—opening doors to progress while upholding human values.

9.3 The Problem of "Stem Cell Tourism"

One of the most significant ethical and safety challenges today is what experts refer to as **stem cell tourism**. This happens when patients—

sometimes out of desperation or hope — visit private, unregulated clinics to receive stem cell treatments that are not approved, not monitored, and not backed by scientific evidence.

These clinics often employ slick marketing tactics, including glossy websites, dramatic before-and-after pictures, and glowing patient testimonials. They may use scientific-sounding language to create the impression of legitimacy. But behind the promises, many of these operations:

- Make **exaggerated claims** about miracle cures.
- Charge patients **tens of thousands of dollars** upfront.
- Operate **without independent oversight** from regulators or ethics boards.
- Offer treatments that **have never been tested** in proper clinical trials.

Sadly, the risks are not only financial. Some patients have experienced severe complications after receiving unproven stem cell injections, including infections, tumor growth, and organ damage. In rare cases, these complications have been life-threatening.

The harm goes beyond individual patients. Stem cell tourism also **undermines public trust in science**. When people hear about adverse outcomes from unregulated clinics, they may become skeptical of stem cell research in general—even when legitimate clinical trials are showing real progress. It can also slow down research, as regulators and scientists must spend time addressing the damage caused by irresponsible clinics.

A Patient's Story: Daniel's Dilemma

Daniel, a 50-year-old engineer, had been battling an aggressive form of lymphoma. After several rounds of treatment, he learned about a private clinic that promised a **"cutting-edge stem cell cure with zero side effects."** The testimonials online sounded convincing, and Daniel was ready to mortgage his home to pay the $35,000 cost.

Daniel shared the clinic's website with his oncologist. She pointed out several red flags: no published data, no registration in a clinical trial database, and vague claims with no scientific detail. Instead, she connected him with a Phase II clinical trial at a cancer center that was testing stem cells in combination with immunotherapy.

Daniel chose the trial. Although it was still experimental, it was **offered free of charge**, carefully monitored, and supported by real science. More importantly, Daniel felt reassured that he was in safe hands. Months later, his scans showed positive signs, but even beyond his own results, he took pride in contributing to research that could help future patients.

Daniel's story shows that asking the right questions and seeking medical guidance can transform desperation into informed hope.

The medical community is clear: **the safest and most hopeful path is through regulated clinical trials**. These trials may move more slowly than flashy clinics, but they are designed to protect patients at every step. By participating in a legitimate trial, patients not only gain access to new therapies safely, but they also help advance science for everyone.

The hopeful message is this: you don't need to travel across the world or empty your savings for a chance at hope. Real progress in stem cell therapies is currently being made in accredited hospitals and research centers. By choosing the safe, evidence-based path, patients protect themselves and contribute to the breakthroughs that will one day make stem cell therapies widely available and trustworthy.

Did You Know?
The **World Health Organization (WHO)** and many cancer societies have issued warnings about unproven stem cell clinics. They remind patients that **legitimate clinical trials are usually free**, and many even help with travel expenses. If a clinic requests tens of thousands of dollars upfront, it is almost certainly not a legitimate trial.

9.4 The Role of Regulation and Oversight

When patients hear about "regulation," they sometimes imagine bureaucracy, red tape, and delays. However, in medicine, regulation exists for one simple reason: **to protect the public**. Stem cell research is a rapidly evolving field, and without proper oversight, unsafe or unproven treatments could reach patients too quickly, causing harm and eroding trust in legitimate scientific research.

Fortunately, there are robust systems in place worldwide to ensure patient safety while still allowing progress to move forward.

- **Ethics Committees and Institutional Review Boards (IRBs)**: These independent groups review every clinical trial before it begins. They check that the study is fair, that patients will give proper informed consent, and that risks are clearly explained. Their role is to ensure that patients are treated with **dignity and respect**.

- **Regulatory Agencies**: Bodies such as the European Medicines Agency (EMA) and the U.S. Food and Drug Administration (FDA) review the scientific evidence behind new stem cell therapies. They decide whether treatments can progress from small, early trials to larger ones, and ultimately whether they can be approved for routine use. This process may feel slow, but it ensures that only therapies with substantial proof of safety and effectiveness reach patients.
- **International Guidelines**: Organizations such as the **International Society for Stem Cell Research (ISSCR)** publish global standards for responsible research. These guidelines shape the operations of labs and clinics in over 80 countries, fostering a shared framework of safety and ethics that transcends borders.

These protective structures may slow things down, but they are the reason that patients can trust approved treatments. They make sure that when a new therapy finally reaches the clinic, it is not just experimental hype—it is a safe, carefully tested option that can genuinely help.

A Patient's Story: Evelyn's Reassurance

Evelyn, a 63-year-old retired nurse, was offered the opportunity to participate in a clinical trial using stem cells to repair tissue damage following chemotherapy. At first, she felt nervous—she had read too many stories about unregulated clinics offering risky treatments for large sums of money.

However, when she learned that the study had been reviewed by an **ethics committee**, registered with **ClinicalTrials.gov**, and approved by the **FDA** to proceed to Phase II, her perspective shifted. Knowing there were multiple layers of oversight gave her confidence. She wasn't stepping into the unknown; she was joining a program that had been carefully evaluated at every step.

Evelyn later shared that the sense of safety and transparency was just as valuable to her as the treatment itself. *"I knew I wasn't being experimented on—I was partnering with a team that put patient protection first. That trust made all the difference."*

The hopeful perspective is this: regulation is not an obstacle to progress—it is what makes progress possible. By keeping patients safe, regulations foster public trust and lay the foundation for stem cell therapies to evolve from promising ideas into everyday cancer treatments.

Did You Know?
The FDA has approved more than **20 cell-based therapies** for blood disorders and immune diseases, with most of these therapies involving stem cells. Every one of these treatments passed through rigorous layers of review—proof that regulation may take time, but it delivers real, lasting results for patients.

9.5 Looking Ahead: Balancing Innovation and Responsibility

Stem cell therapies sit at the edge of one of medicine's most exciting frontiers. Scientists, doctors, and patients all share the same hope: that these remarkable cells will one day help us not only treat cancer more effectively but also repair the damage left behind by harsh therapies. However, as with every frontier, the path forward must strike a balance between two equally important goals: **innovation** and **responsibility**.

- **Innovation** means pushing science to its limits—finding new ways to engineer stem cells, combining them with cutting-edge tools like immunotherapy and CRISPR, and testing bold ideas that could one day cure diseases that seem impossible to treat today.
- **Responsibility** means making sure these innovations are developed safely, ethically, and fairly. Patients must never be treated as experiments without consent, and breakthroughs must not be limited only to those who can afford them.

Striking this balance is not easy. Excessive caution can hinder progress and delay access to treatments that patients desperately need. Too little caution risks exposing vulnerable people to harm. The challenge for researchers, regulators, and healthcare systems is to walk the middle path: moving forward as quickly as possible, but never at the expense of patient safety or dignity.

Encouragingly, the global community is already rising to this challenge. International guidelines, national oversight bodies, and patient advocacy groups are shaping a future where stem cell therapies are developed with **both speed and safety**. Scientists themselves often emphasize that building patient trust through transparency is as important as the discoveries happening in the lab.

The most hopeful truth is this: ethical responsibility and scientific innovation are not enemies—they are partners. By protecting patients today, we lay the groundwork for building trust, knowledge, and a foundation that will make stem cell therapies a routine part of cancer care tomorrow.

Did You Know?
Bone marrow transplants, once seen as risky and experimental, are now a **standard treatment for blood cancers worldwide.** This transformation demonstrates how responsible research, conducted in a step-by-step manner, can transform what seems uncertain today into lifesaving therapies for millions.

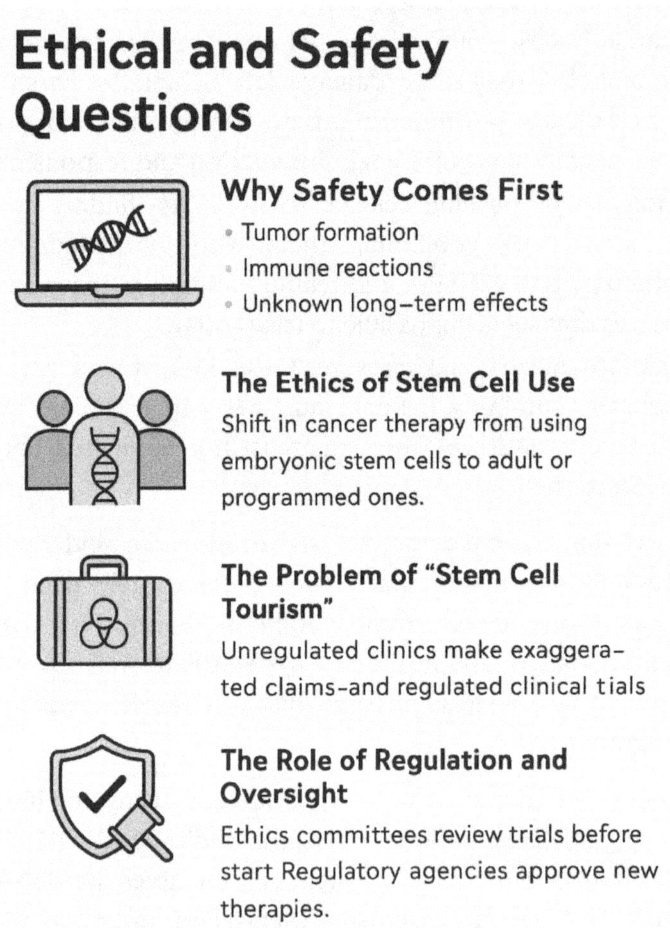

Ethical and Safety Questions
Why Safety Comes First
• Tumor formation
• Immune reactions
• Unknown long-term effects
The Ethics of Stem Cell Use
Shift in cancer therapy from using embryonic stem cells to adult or programmed ones.
The Problem of "Stem Cell Tourism"
Unregulated clinics make exaggera-ted claims-and regulated clinical tials
The Role of Regulation and Oversight
Ethics committees review trials before start Regulatory agencies approve new therapies.

Chapter 10 – The Future of Stem Cells in Cancer Therapy

Stem cell research is one of the most dynamic and fast-moving areas of modern medicine. What once sounded like science fiction—using the body's own "master cells" to fight cancer and repair damage—is now entering real-world clinical trials. The question is no longer *"Will stem cells change cancer care?"* but rather *"How, and how soon?"*

This final chapter looks ahead, exploring the most promising directions, the challenges that remain, and why patients and families have real reason to feel hopeful about the future.

> ***Patient Quote:*** *"When my granddaughter asked if cancer would always be this scary, I told her, ' Not forever. With new research, maybe her generation will see a world where stem cell therapies make cancer easier to treat."* — Evelyn, 67.

10.1 Promising Directions in Research

Scientists are finding increasingly creative ways to use stem cells in cancer therapy. Some of the most promising directions include:

- **Smarter Stem Cells**: Engineered stem cells can act like targeted couriers, delivering chemotherapy, immune-boosting signals, or even genetic tools directly into tumors. This approach could make treatments both more powerful and less toxic.
- **Immune System Allies**: Stem cells may one day act as "teachers" for the immune system, training T cells and other defenders to recognize and attack even the most hidden cancer cells.
- **Repair and Recovery**: Beyond destroying tumors, stem cells may also help rebuild what cancer and its treatments have damaged—repairing bone marrow, regenerating tissue, and reducing long-term side effects.

These possibilities show that stem cells are not just about fighting cancer, but also about helping patients heal and live better after treatment.

Did You Know?
In some early trials, mesenchymal stem cells (MSCs) have already been tested to reduce damage from radiation therapy—helping heal tissues such as the intestines, skin, and salivary glands.

10.2 Personalized Medicine

No two cancers are exactly alike. Each tumor has its own "genetic fingerprint," which explains why some treatments work for one patient but not for another.

The future of stem cell therapy is pointing toward **personalized medicine**—designing treatments that are tailor-made for each individual:

- Doctors may one day take a patient's own stem cells, reprogram them in the lab, and send them back as a custom therapy targeted to that patient's exact tumor mutations.
- Advances in **genetic sequencing** and **artificial intelligence** could help doctors match patients to the most effective stem cell therapies, avoiding one-size-fits-all approaches.

Personalization means fewer side effects, more targeted results, and a future where cancer care feels less like trial-and-error and more like precision science.

> ***A Patient's Story: Maya's Window into the Future*** - Maya, a 39-year-old scientist diagnosed with breast cancer, participated in a study that sequenced her tumor's DNA. While standard chemotherapy was recommended, she was also shown a preview of how, in the near future, her own stem cells might be engineered to attack the specific mutations in her cancer. For Maya, knowing that science was moving toward highly personalized treatments gave her hope—not just for herself, but for her children's generation.

10.3 Combining Stem Cells with Other Innovations

Stem cells will not be working alone in the future of cancer care. Instead, they are likely to be part of a **team effort** alongside other groundbreaking technologies:

- **Immunotherapy**: Boosting the body's natural defenses while stem cells help deliver or reinforce the fight.

- **CRISPR Gene Editing**: Allowing scientists to "recode" stem cells for greater precision, resistance to cancer, or enhanced immune support.
- **Nanotechnology**: Loading stem cells with ultra-small particles that can release drugs exactly where they are needed inside a tumor.

Together, these tools could create treatments that are **more powerful, more targeted, and longer-lasting** than anything we have today.

Did You Know?
In 2020, the first patients received **CRISPR-edited immune cells** in a clinical trial for cancer. Early results showed the approach was safe—opening the door to combining CRISPR with stem cell therapy in the near future.

10.4 Overcoming Challenges

The path forward is bright, but challenges remain:

- **Safety**: Scientists must ensure that engineered stem cells do not cause unintended problems, such as the formation of new tumors.
- **Accessibility**: Cutting-edge therapies risk being available only in wealthy countries or to patients who can afford high costs. Ensuring fairness will be critical.
- **Regulation**: Clear rules must be in place to enable innovation while maintaining patient safety.

History gives us reason to be hopeful. Bone marrow transplants, once seen as risky and controversial, are now standard care for thousands of cancer patients worldwide. Step by step, careful science has turned yesterday's experimental ideas into today's lifesaving treatments.

The same journey is happening now with stem cell therapies.

Did You Know?
More than **400 clinical trials** worldwide are currently testing stem cell–based cancer therapies. Each trial adds to the knowledge base, bringing us closer to safe and effective treatments for millions.

10.5 A Future of Hope

The story of stem cells in cancer is still being written—but each chapter brings us closer to a brighter ending. Stem cell therapies are not a magic bullet, but they hold the potential to **transform cancer care**: making treatments more effective, less toxic, and more personal.

For patients and their families, the message is clear: hope is not only on the horizon—it is already underway.

✨ *Every clinical trial, every patient who participates, and every breakthrough in the lab moves us closer to a world where cancer is not a life sentence, but a disease that can be managed—and perhaps one day cured.*

💬 Patient Takeaway – Looking Ahead with Hope

"What feels experimental today may be the treatment that saves lives tomorrow. By moving carefully but boldly, science is bringing us closer to a future where stem cells not only fight cancer but also help patients heal and thrive."

✨ The partnership of innovation and responsibility is building a future of medicine that is safer, smarter, and full of promise.

The Future of Stem Cells in Cancer Therapy

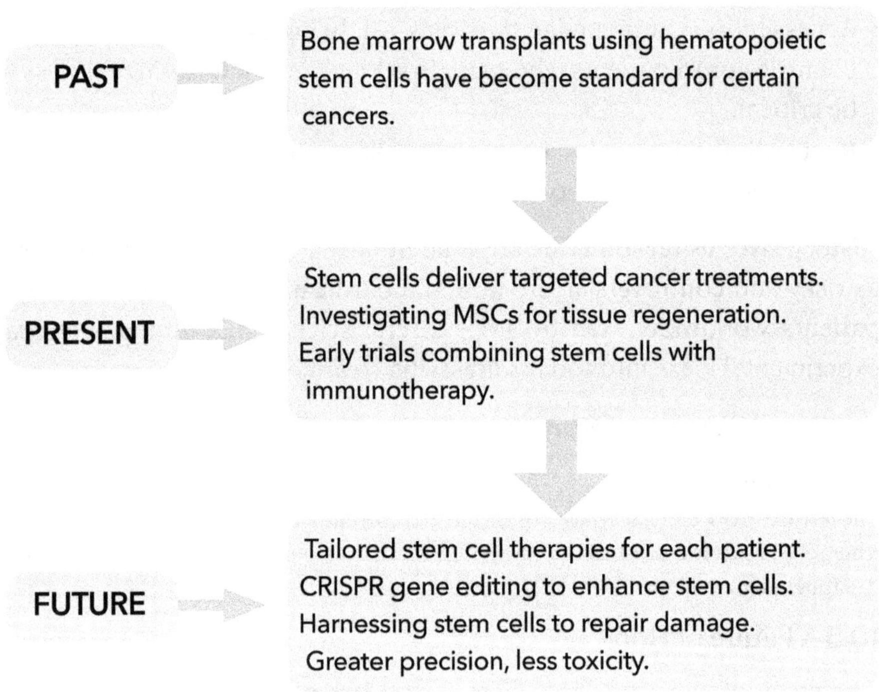

Author

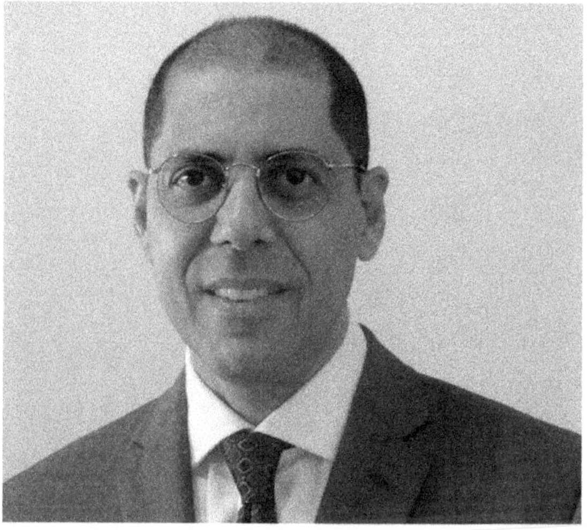

Dr. Marcio Alvarez-Silva is a university professor specializing in Cellular Biology and Cancer Biology. He has served on the editorial boards of several scientific journals, including:

1. MAYFEB Journal of Medicine (2016–2018)

2. International Journal of Pathology and Clinical Research (2015–present)

3. Current Stem Cell Research & Therapy (2019–present)

Dr. Alvarez-Silva has authored articles in peer-reviewed journals and contributed to books on oncology, such as:

-"Stem Cell Niche and Microenvironment," in *Principles of Stem Cell Biology and Cancer: Future Applications and Therapeutics* (Wiley-Blackwell)

- *Under the Sign of Cancer: Learn More About the History, Prevention, and Treatment of Cancer* (Direct Publishing)

In March 2019, he founded the digital magazine Understanding Cancer (https://en.ucancer.org/), providing comprehensive information on cancer and related therapies.

References

1. Slack, J.M.W., *Stem Cells in Epithelial Tissues.* Science, 2000. **287** (5457): p. 1431-1433.

2. Remak, R., *Untersuchungen über die Entwickelung der Wirbelthiere.* 1855, Berlin: G. Reimer. 194.

3. Virchow, R., *Die Cellularpathologie.* 1858, Berlin: Verlag von August Hirschwald. 444.

4. Hyun, I., *The bioethics of stem cell research and therapy.* The Journal of Clinical Investigation, 2010. **120** (1): p. 71-75.

5. National Institutes of Health. *Stem Cell Basics.* Available from: https://stemcells.nih.gov/info/basics.

6. Friedenstein, A.J., R.K. Chailakhjan, and K.S. Lalykina, *The development of fibroblast colonies in monolayer cultures of guinea-pig bone marrow and spleen cells.* Cell Proliferation, 1970. **3** (4): p. 393-403.

7. Erices, A., P. Conget, and J.J. Minguell, *Mesenchymal progenitor cells in human umbilical cord blood.* British Journal of Haematology, 2000. **109** (1): p. 235-242.

8. Gronthos, S., et al., *Postnatal human dental pulp stem cells (DPSCs) in vitro and in vivo.* Proceedings of the National Academy of Sciences, 2000. **97** (25): p. 13625-13630.

9. Zuk, P.A., et al., *Human Adipose Tissue Is a Source of Multipotent Stem Cells.* Molecular Biology of the Cell, 2002. **13** (12): p. 4279-4295.

10. Fukuchi, Y., et al., *Human Placenta-Derived Cells Have Mesenchymal Stem/Progenitor Cell Potential.* Stem Cells, 2004. **22** (5): p. 649-658.

11. Wang, H.S., et al., *Mesenchymal Stem Cells in the Wharton's Jelly of the*

Human Umbilical Cord. Stem Cells, 2004. **22** (7): p. 1330-1337.

12. Paul, G., et al., *The Adult Human Brain Harbors Multipotent Perivascular Mesenchymal Stem Cells.* PLOS ONE, 2012. **7** (4): p. e35577.

13. Lai, R.C., R.W.Y. Yeo, and S.K. Lim, *Mesenchymal stem cell exosomes.* Seminars in Cell & Developmental Biology, 2015. **40**: p. 82-88.

14. Pittenger, M.F., et al., *Multilineage Potential of Adult Human Mesenchymal Stem Cells.* Science, 1999. **284** (5411): p. 143-147.

15. Bianco, P., *Bone and the hematopoietic niche: a tale of two stem cells.* Blood, 2011. **117** (20): p. 5281-5288.

16. Marconi, G.D., et al., *Three-Dimensional Culture System: A New Frontier in Cancer Research, Drug Discovery, and Stem Cell-Based Therapy.* Biology, 2025. **14** (7): p. 875.

17. Nittayaboon, K., et al., *Bone Marrow Mesenchymal Stem Cell-Derived Exosomes Modulate Chemoradiotherapy Response in Cervical Cancer Spheroids.* Pharmaceuticals, 2025. **18** (7): p. 1050.

18. Shokati, A., et al., *Revolutionizing cancer treatment: engineering mesenchymal stem cell-derived small extracellular vesicles.* Cancer Cell International, 2025. **25** (1): p. 275.

19. Thomas, E.D., *Bone marrow transplantation: past, present and future.* Rev Invest Clin, 1994. **Suppl**: p. 5-6.

20. Alvarez-Silva, M., *Advances in Hematopoietic Stem Cell Transplantation.* Advanced Techniques in Biology & Medicine, 2017. **5** (1): p. 210-214.

21. Takahashi, K. and S. Yamanaka, *Induction of pluripotent stem cells from mouse embryonic and adult fibroblast cultures by defined factors.* Cell, 2006. **126** (4): p. 663-76.

22. Thomas, E.D., et al., *Intravenous Infusion of Bone Marrow in Patients Receiving Radiation and Chemotherapy.* New England Journal of Medicine, 1957. **257** (11): p. 491-496.

23. Del Papa, N., et al., *Autologous Hematopoietic Stem Cell Transplantation for Treatment of Systemic Sclerosis.* Frontiers in Immunology, 2018. **Volume 9 - 2018**.

24. Balassa, K., R. Danby, and V. Rocha, *Haematopoietic stem cell transplants: principles and indications.* British Journal of Hospital Medicine, 2019. **80** (1):

p. 33-39.

25. Bazinet, A. and G. Popradi, *A General Practitioner's Guide to Hematopoietic Stem-cell Transplantation.* Current Oncology, 2019. **26** (3): p. 187-191.

26. Rostami, T., et al., *Hematopoietic Stem Cell Transplantation in Sickle Cell Disease: A Multidimentional Review.* Cell Transplantation, 2024. **33**: p. 09636897241246351.

27. Zuk, P.A., et al., *Multilineage cells from human adipose tissue: implications for cell-based therapies.* Tissue Eng, 2001. **7** (2): p. 211-28.

28. Weiss, M.L., et al., *Human Umbilical Cord Matrix Stem Cells: Preliminary Characterization and Effect of Transplantation in a Rodent Model of Parkinson's Disease.* Stem Cells, 2005. **24** (3): p. 781-792.

29. Coura, G.S., et al., *Human periodontal ligament: a niche of neural crest stem cells.* J Periodontal Res, 2008. **43** (5): p. 531-6.

30. Martini, M.M., et al., *Human placenta-derived mesenchymal stem cells acquire neural phenotype under the appropriate niche conditions.* DNA and Cell Biology, 2013. **32** (2): p. 58-65.

31. Xu, X., et al., *Harnessing knee joint resident mesenchymal stem cells in cartilage tissue engineering.* Acta Biomaterialia, 2023. **168**: p. 372-387.

32. Jiang, Y., et al., *Amniotic Fluid-Derived Stem Cells: An Overlooked Source of Stem Cells for Translational Research.* DNA and Cell Biology, 2025. **44** (3): p. 144-152.

33. Dominici, M., et al., *Minimal criteria for defining multipotent mesenchymal stromal cells. The International Society for Cellular Therapy position statement.* Cytotherapy, 2006. **8** (4): p. 315-317.

34. Glennie, S., et al., *Bone marrow mesenchymal stem cells induce division arrest anergy of activated T cells.* Blood, 2005. **105** (7): p. 2821-2827.

35. Phinney, D.G. and M.F. Pittenger, *Concise Review: MSC-Derived Exosomes for Cell-Free Therapy.* Stem Cells, 2017. **35** (4): p. 851-858.

36. Hass, R., et al., *Different populations and sources of human mesenchymal stem cells (MSC): A comparison of adult and neonatal tissue-derived MSC.* Cell Communication and Signaling, 2011. **9** (1): p. 12.

37. Reya, T., et al., *Stem cells, cancer, and cancer stem cells.* Nature, 2001. **414** (6859): p. 105-111.

38. Ikonomou, L., et al., *International Society for Cell & Gene Therapy Position Paper: Key considerations to support evidence-based cell and gene therapies and oppose marketing of unproven products.* Cytotherapy, 2023. **25** (9): p. 920-929.

39. Schüz, J., et al., *European Code against Cancer 4th Edition: 12 ways to reduce your cancer risk.* Cancer Epidemiology, 2015. **39**: p. S1-S10.

40. Falzone, L., et al., *Occupational exposure to carcinogens: Benzene, pesticides and fibers (Review).* Molecular Medicine Reports, 2016. **14** (5): p. 4467-4474.

41. American Cancer Society. *Cancer Risk Factors.* Available from: https://www.cancer.org/healthy/cancer-causes.html.

42. *Cancer Causes and Risk Factors.* Available from: https://www.cancer.gov/about-cancer/causes-prevention.

43. Hanahan, D. and R.A. Weinberg, *The Hallmarks of Cancer.* Cell, 2000. **100** (1): p. 57-70.

44. Hanahan, D. and Robert A. Weinberg, *Hallmarks of Cancer: The Next Generation.* Cell, 2011. **144** (5): p. 646-674.

45. Floor, S.L., et al., *Hallmarks of cancer: of all cancer cells, all the time?* Trends in Molecular Medicine, 2012. **18** (9): p. 509-515.

46. Levine, A.J. and M. Oren, *The first 30 years of p53: growing ever more complex.* Nat Rev Cancer, 2009. **9** (10): p. 749-58.

47. Batlle, E. and H. Clevers, *Cancer stem cells revisited.* Nature Medicine, 2017. **23** (10): p. 1124-1134.

48. World Health Organization – International Agency for Research on Cancer. Available from: https://www.iarc.who.int.

49. Dean, M., T. Fojo, and S. Bates, *Tumour stem cells and drug resistance.* Nature Reviews Cancer, 2005. **5** (4): p. 275-284.

50. Visvader, J.E. and G.J. Lindeman, *Cancer stem cells in solid tumours: accumulating evidence and unresolved questions.* Nat Rev Cancer, 2008. **8** (10): p. 755-768.

51. Phi, L.T.H., et al., *Cancer Stem Cells (CSCs) in Drug Resistance and their Therapeutic Implications in Cancer Treatment.* Stem Cells International, 2018. **2018** (1): p. 5416923.

52. Keith, B. and M.C. Simon, *Hypoxia-Inducible Factors, Stem Cells, and Cancer.* Cell, 2007. **129** (3): p. 465-472.

53. Gonzalez, H., C. Hagerling, and Z. Werb, *Roles of the immune system in cancer: from tumor initiation to metastatic progression.* Genes Dev, 2018. **32** (19-20): p. 1267-1284.

54. Takebe, N., et al., *Targeting Notch, Hedgehog, and Wnt pathways in cancer stem cells: clinical update.* Nature Reviews Clinical Oncology, 2015. **12** (8): p. 445-464.

55. Clevers, H., *Modeling Development and Disease with Organoids.* Cell, 2016. **165** (7): p. 1586-1597.

56. Copelan , E.A., *Hematopoietic Stem-Cell Transplantation.* New England Journal of Medicine, 2006. **354** (17): p. 1813-1826.

57. Studeny, M., et al., *Mesenchymal Stem Cells: Potential Precursors for Tumor Stroma and Targeted-Delivery Vehicles for Anticancer Agents.* JNCI: Journal of the National Cancer Institute, 2004. **96** (21): p. 1593-1603.

58. Loebinger, M.R., et al., *Mesenchymal Stem Cell Delivery of TRAIL Can Eliminate Metastatic Cancer.* Cancer Research, 2009. **69** (10): p. 4134-4142.

59. Themeli, M., et al., *Generation of tumor-targeted human T lymphocytes from induced pluripotent stem cells for cancer therapy.* Nature Biotechnology, 2013. **31** (10): p. 928-933.

60. Sachs, N., et al., *A Living Biobank of Breast Cancer Organoids Captures Disease Heterogeneity.* Cell, 2018. **172** (1): p. 373-386.e10.

61. Doudna, J.A. and E. Charpentier, *The new frontier of genome engineering with CRISPR-Cas9.* Science, 2014. **346** (6213): p. 1258096.

62. Akbari Kordkheyli, V., et al., *CRISPER/CAS System, a Novel Tool of Targeted Therapy of Drug-Resistant Lung Cancer.* Adv Pharm Bull, 2022. **12** (2): p. 262-273.

63. Gragert, L., et al., *HLA match likelihoods for hematopoietic stem-cell grafts in the U.S. registry.* N Engl J Med, 2014. **371** (4): p. 339-48.

64. Alseraihy, A., et al., *Worldwide Network for Blood and Marrow Transplantation Special Article on Key Elements in Quality and Accreditation in Hematopoietic Stem Cell Transplantation and Cellular Therapy.* Transplantation and Cellular Therapy, 2022. **28** (8): p. 455-462.

65. Kurtzberg, J., et al., *Unrelated Donor Cord Blood Transplantation in Children:*

Lessons Learned Over 3 Decades. Stem Cells Translational Medicine, 2023. **12** (1): p. 26-38.

66. Dever, D.P., et al., *CRISPR/Cas9 β-globin gene targeting in human haematopoietic stem cells*. Nature, 2016. **539** (7629): p. 384-389.

67. Mozaffari Jovein, M., et al., *Long-term follow-up of patients with acute myeloid leukemia undergoing allogeneic hematopoietic stem cell transplantation after primary induction failure*. Blood Cancer Journal, 2023. **13** (1): p. 179.

68. Tan, E.H.P., et al., *Perspectives on the use and availability of chimeric antigen receptor T cells (CAR-T) and cell therapies: A worldwide cross-sectional survey by the worldwide network for blood and marrow transplantation (WBMT)*. Current Research in Translational Medicine, 2025. **73** (2): p. 103515.

69. Alousi, A. and M. de Lima, *Reduced-intensity conditioning allogeneic hematopoietic stem cell transplantation*. Clin Adv Hematol Oncol, 2007. **5** (7): p. 560-70.

70. Gyurkocza, B. and B.M. Sandmaier, *Conditioning regimens for hematopoietic cell transplantation: one size does not fit all*. Blood, 2014. **124** (3): p. 344-353.

71. Passweg, J.R., et al., *Utilization of hematopoietic cell transplantation and cellular therapy technology in Europe and associated Countries. Using the 2022 activity survey data to correlate with economic and demographic factors. A report from the EBMT*. Bone Marrow Transplantation, 2025. **60** (2): p. 227-236.

72. Jimenez Jimenez, A.M., et al., *Allogeneic Hematopoietic Cell Donor Selection: Contemporary Guidelines from the NMDP/CIBMTR*. Transplantation and Cellular Therapy, 2025.

73. Pineault, N. and A. Abu-Khader, *Advances in umbilical cord blood stem cell expansion and clinical translation*. Experimental Hematology, 2015. **43** (7): p. 498-513.

74. Hong, S. and M.E. Horwitz, *Graft Source Choice*, in *Clinical Management of Challenges in Allogeneic Stem Cell Transplant*, K. Ballen, Editor. 2025, Springer Nature Switzerland: Cham. p. 57-75.

75. McManus, M., H. Frangoul, and M.H. Steinberg, *CRISPR-based gene therapy for the induction of fetal hemoglobin in sickle cell disease*. Expert Review of Hematology, 2024. **17** (12): p. 957-966.

76. Levesque, S. and D.E. Bauer, *CRISPR-based therapeutic genome editing for inherited blood disorders* Nature Reviews Drug Discovery, 2025.

77. Saccardi, R., et al., *Benchmarking of survival outcomes following Haematopoietic Stem Cell Transplantation (HSCT): an update of the ongoing project of the European Society for Blood and Marrow Transplantation (EBMT) and Joint Accreditation Committee of ISCT and EBMT (JACIE).* Bone Marrow Transplantation, 2023. **58** (6): p. 659-666.

78. Atsuta, Y., et al., *Continuous and differential improvement in worldwide access to hematopoietic cell transplantation: activity has doubled in a decade with a notable increase in unrelated and non-identical related donors.* Haematologica, 2024. **109** (10): p. 3282-3294.

79. National Cancer Institute. *Three-Drug Regimen Improves Protection against GVHD after Stem Cell Transplant.* Available from: https://www.cancer.gov/news-events/cancer-currents-blog/2023/gvhd-prevention-stem-cell-transplant-cyclophosphamide?utm_source=chatgpt.com.

80. Dana-Farber Cancer Institute. *What's New in Prevention and Treatment of Chronic GVHD.* Available from: https://www.dana-farber.org/for-physicians/clinical-resources/hematologic-malignancies/advances-newsletter/2024-issue-19/chronic-gvhd?utm_source=chatgpt.com.

81. Shah, R., et al., *Multidisciplinary Management of Morbidities Associated with Chronic Graft-Versus-Host Disease.* Clin Hematol Int, 2024. **6** (4): p. 74-88.

82. Silva-Pinto, A., et al., *Vaccination After Haematopoietic Stem Cell Transplant: A Review of the Literature and Proposed Vaccination Protocol.* Vaccines (Basel), 2024. **12** (12).

83. Savaş, E.M., et al., *COVID-19 Vaccine Response in Allo-HSCT Recipients: Insights from a Real-World Prospective Cohort Study.* Vaccines, 2025. **13** (7): p. 726.

84. Epstein, D.J., et al., *Infectious Disease Considerations in Chronic Graft-versus-Host Disease and Transplantation Survivors.* Transplantation and Cellular Therapy, Official Publication of the American Society for Transplantation and Cellular Therapy, 2024. **30** (9): p. S534-S547.

85. Bouzas-Rodríguez, A., et al., *Vaccination Coverage in Hematopoietic Stem Cell Transplant Patients.* Vaccines, 2025. **13** (3): p. 257.

86. Figueiredo, C. and R. Blasczyk, *A future with less HLA: potential clinical*

applications of HLA-universal cells. Tissue Antigens, 2015. **85** (6): p. 443-449.

87. Bertaina, A. and M.G. Roncarolo, *Graft Engineering and Adoptive Immunotherapy: New Approaches to Promote Immune Tolerance After Hematopoietic Stem Cell Transplantation.* Frontiers in Immunology, 2019. **Volume 10 - 2019**.

88. Simpson, A., A.W. Hewitt, and K.A. Fairfax, *Universal cell donor lines: A review of the current research.* Stem Cell Reports, 2023. **18** (11): p. 2038-2046.

89. Thangavelu, G., et al., *Chapter 17 - Insights and strategies to promote immune tolerance in allogeneic hematopoietic stem cell transplantation recipients,* in *Translational Autoimmunity,* N. Rezaei, Editor. 2023, Academic Press. p. 329-360.

90. Tsiverioti, C.A., et al., *Beyond CAR T cells: exploring alternative cell sources for CAR-like cellular therapies.* Biological Chemistry, 2024. **405** (7-8): p. 485-515.

91. Mishra, H.K. and A. Kalyuzhny, *Revolutionizing Cancer Treatments through Stem Cell-Derived CAR T Cells for Immunotherapy: Opening New Horizons for the Future of Oncology.* Cells, 2024. **13** (18): p. 1516.

92. Li, L.-L., et al., *Case report: CD7-targeted autologous CAR-T therapy for the treatment of T-cell acute lymphoblastic leukemia undergoing allogeneic peripheral blood stem cell transplantation in the long-term follow-up.* Frontiers in Immunology, 2024. **Volume 15 - 2024**.

93. Zhang, C., et al., *Long-term survival with donor CD19 CAR-T cell treatment for relapsed patients after allogeneic hematopietic stem cell transplantation.* Journal of Hematology & Oncology, 2024. **17** (1): p. 103.

94. Zimran, E., L. Papa, and R. Hoffman, *Ex vivo expansion of hematopoietic stem cells: Finally transitioning from the lab to the clinic.* Blood Reviews, 2021. **50**: p. 100853.

95. Saiyin, T., et al., *Clinical Outcomes of Umbilical Cord Blood Transplantation Using Ex Vivo Expansion: A Systematic Review and Meta-Analysis of Controlled Studies.* Transplantation and Cellular Therapy, Official Publication of the American Society for Transplantation and Cellular Therapy, 2023. **29** (2): p. 129.e1-129.e9.

96. Branco, A., et al., *Advances in ex vivo expansion of hematopoietic stem and progenitor cells for clinical applications.* Frontiers in Bioengineering and

Biotechnology, 2024. **Volume 12 - 2024**.

97. Hooijmaijers, L., et al., *Good manufacturing practice production of an off-the-shelf CD34+ progenitor-derived NK cell product with preserved anti-tumor functionality post-infusion in NOD/SCID/IL2Rgnull mice.* Cellular and Molecular Life Sciences, 2025. **82** (1): p. 210.

98. Strati, P., et al., *Off-the-shelf induced pluripotent stem-cell-derived natural killer-cell therapy in relapsed or refractory B-cell lymphoma: a multicentre, open-label, phase 1 study.* The Lancet Haematology, 2025. **12** (7): p. e505-e515.

99. Pittenger, M.F., et al., *MSCs: Scientific Support for Multiple Therapies.* Stem Cells International, 2015. **2015**: p. 2.

100. Ho, Y.K., et al., *Enhanced anti-tumor efficacy with multi-transgene armed mesenchymal stem cells for treating peritoneal carcinomatosis.* Journal of Translational Medicine, 2024. **22** (1): p. 463.

101. Shi, Y., et al., *Engineered mesenchymal stem/stromal cells against cancer.* Cell Death & Disease, 2025. **16** (1): p. 113.

102. Alvarez-Silva, M., *Stem Cell Niche and Microenvironment,* in *Principles of Stem Cell Biology and Cancer*. 2015, John Wiley & Sons, Ltd. p. 45-64.

103. Ding, Y., et al., *Mesenchymal Stem Cells Engineered by Nonviral Vectors: A Powerful Tool in Cancer Gene Therapy.* Pharmaceutics, 2021. **13** (6): p. 913.

104. Shams, F., et al., *Current progress in engineered and nano-engineered mesenchymal stem cells for cancer: From mechanisms to therapy.* Biomedicine & Pharmacotherapy, 2023. **167**: p. 115505.

105. Garza Treviño, E.N., et al., *Applications of Modified Mesenchymal Stem Cells as Targeted Systems against Tumor Cells.* International Journal of Molecular Sciences, 2024. **25** (14): p. 7791.

106. TomyTomcy, A. and E.R. Sindhu, *Mesenchymal stem cells- an excellent therapeutic agent for cancer.* Asia-Pacific Journal of Clinical Oncology, 2024. **20** (1): p. 7-15.

107. ClinicalTrials.gov. *Studies on mesenchymal stem cells and cancer.* Available from: https://clinicaltrials.gov.

108. Spaeth, E.L., et al., *Mesenchymal stem cell transition to tumor-associated fibroblasts contributes to fibrovascular network expansion and tumor progression.* PLoS ONE, 2009. **4**.

109. Kucerova, L., et al., *Cytosine deaminase expressing human mesenchymal stem cells mediated tumour regression in melanoma bearing mice.* The Journal of Gene Medicine, 2008. **10** (10): p. 1071-1082.

110. Sarkisova, V.A., et al., *Cell Carriers for Oncolytic Virus Delivery: Prospects for Systemic Administration.* Cancers, 2025. **17** (14): p. 2296.

111. Vogiatzi, I., et al., *Allogeneic stem cells engineered to release interferon β and scFv-PD1 target glioblastoma and alter the tumor microenvironment.* Cytotherapy, 2024. **26** (10): p. 1217-1226.

112. Razeghian, E., et al., *Mesenchymal Stem/Stromal Cells as a Vehicle for Cytokine Delivery: An Emerging Approach for Tumor Immunotherapy.* Front Med (Lausanne), 2021. **8**: p. 721174.

113. Mehralizadeh, H., et al., *Cytokine sustained delivery for cancer therapy; special focus on stem cell- and biomaterial- based delivery methods.* Pathology - Research and Practice, 2023. **247**: p. 154528.

114. The Source - Washington University. *Innovative immunotherapy shows promise against aggressive T cell cancers.* Available from: https://source.washu.edu/2025/05/innovative-immunotherapy-shows-promise-against-aggressive-t-cell-cancers/?utm_source=chatgpt.com.

115. Alali, Z., et al., *Stem Cell for Cancer Immunotherapy: Current Approaches and Challenges.* Stem Cell Reviews and Reports, 2025.

116. Mathan, S.V. and R.P. Singh, *Cancer Stem Cells Connecting to Immunotherapy: Key Insights, Challenges, and Potential Treatment Opportunities.* Cancers, 2025. **17** (13): p. 2100.

117. Zhai, R., et al., *Comparative Analysis of the Therapeutic Effects of MSCs From Umbilical Cord, Bone Marrow, and Adipose Tissue and Investigating the Impact of Oxidized RNA on Radiation-Induced Lung Injury.* Stem Cells International, 2024. **2024** (1): p. 7419270.

118. Fenger Carlander, A.-L., et al., *Long-term Effectiveness and Safety of Mesenchymal Stromal Cell Therapy for Radiation-Induced Hyposalivation in Head and Neck Cancer Survivors: A Randomized Phase II Trial.* Clinical Cancer Research, 2025. **31** (5): p. 824-831.

119. Zanoni, M., et al., *The Role of Mesenchymal Stem Cells in Radiation-Induced Lung Fibrosis.* International Journal of Molecular Sciences, 2019. **20** (16): p. 3876.

120. Zeinalzadeh, F., et al., *The role of mesenchymal stem cells and their exosomes in radiotherapy: A new opportunity or a potential threat.* Biochimica et Biophysica Acta (BBA) - General Subjects, 2025. **1869** (8): p. 130823.

121. Mirage News. *IAEA Begins Stem Cell Project for Radiation Injuries.* Available from: https://www.miragenews.com/iaea-begins-stem-cell-project-for-radiation-1509455/?utm_source=chatgpt.com.

122. Chu, X., et al., *Cancer stem cells: advances in knowledge and implications for cancer therapy.* Signal Transduction and Targeted Therapy, 2024. **9** (1): p. 170.

123. Bose, B., U. Sen, and S. Shenoy P, *Breast Cancer Stem Cell Therapeutics, Multiple Strategies Versus Using Engineered Mesenchymal Stem Cells With Notch Inhibitory Properties: Possibilities and Perspectives.* Journal of Cellular Biochemistry, 2018. **119** (1): p. 141-149.

124. Xu, Y., et al., *Endometrium-derived mesenchymal stem cells suppress progression of endometrial cancer via the DKK1-Wnt/β-catenin signaling pathway.* Stem Cell Research & Therapy, 2023. **14** (1): p. 159.

125. Volarevic, V., et al., *Mesenchymal stem cell-derived factors: Immuno-modulatory effects and therapeutic potential.* BioFactors, 2017. **43** (5): p. 633-644.

126. Tang, J., et al., *The role of mesenchymal stem cells in cancer and prospects for their use in cancer therapeutics.* MedComm, 2024. **5** (8): p. e663.

127. Najar, M., et al., *Mesenchymal stromal cells and immunomodulation: A gathering of regulatory immune cells.* Cytotherapy, 2016. **18** (2): p. 160-171.

128. Rosu, A., et al., *Tumor-tropic Trojan horses: Using mesenchymal stem cells as cellular nanotheranostics.* Theranostics, 2024. **14** (2): p. 571-591.

129. Shah, S. and B. Lucke-Wold, *Image-Guided Mesenchymal Stem Cell Sodium Iodide Symporter (NIS) Radionuclide Therapy for Glioblastoma.* Cancers, 2024. **16** (16): p. 2892.

130. Minev, T., et al., *Mesenchymal stem cells - the secret agents of cancer immunotherapy: Promises, challenges, and surprising twists.* Oncotarget, 2024. **15**: p. 793-805.

131. Lu, W. and J. Allickson, *Mesenchymal stromal cell therapy: Progress to date and future outlook.* Molecular Therapy, 2025. **33** (6): p. 2679-2688.

132. Hussen, B.M., et al., *Revolutionizing medicine: recent developments and future prospects in stem-cell therapy.* Int J Surg, 2024. **110** (12): p. 8002-8024.

133. Patel, J.C., M. Shukla, and M. Shukla, *From bench to bedside: translating mesenchymal stem cell therapies through preclinical and clinical evidence.* Frontiers in Bioengineering and Biotechnology, 2025. **Volume 13 - 2025**.

134. Kim, J.-H., et al., *Perspectives on the cost of goods for hPSC banks for manufacture of cell therapies.* npj Regenerative Medicine, 2022. **7** (1): p. 54.

135. Diederichs, S., K.M. Shine, and R.S. Tuan, *The promise and challenges of stem cell-based therapies for skeletal diseases.* BioEssays, 2013. **35** (3): p. 220-230.

136. de Almeida Fuzeta, M., et al., *Addressing the Manufacturing Challenges of Cell-Based Therapies*, in *Current Applications of Pharmaceutical Biotechnology*, A.C. Silva, et al., Editors. 2020, Springer International Publishing: Cham. p. 225-278.

137. Stadtmauer, E.A., et al., *CRISPR-engineered T cells in patients with refractory cancer.* Science, 2020. **367** (6481): p. eaba7365.

138. Ballen, K.K., E. Gluckman, and H.E. Broxmeyer, *Umbilical cord blood transplantation: the first 25 years and beyond.* Vol. 122. 2013. 491-498.

139. Le Blanc, K., et al., *Mesenchymal stem cells for treatment of steroid-resistant, severe, acute graft-versus-host disease: a phase II study.* The Lancet, 2008. **371** (9624): p. 1579-1586.

140. American Cancer Society. *Understanding Cancer.* Available from: https://www.cancer.org/cancer/cancer-basics/what-is-cancer.html.

www.ingramcontent.com/pod-product-compliance
Lightning Source LLC
Chambersburg PA
CBHW071350230926
51846CB00002B/498